Dr. Bell,

It was very good to meet you!

I look forward to further exploring opportunities to collaborate with you and your team!

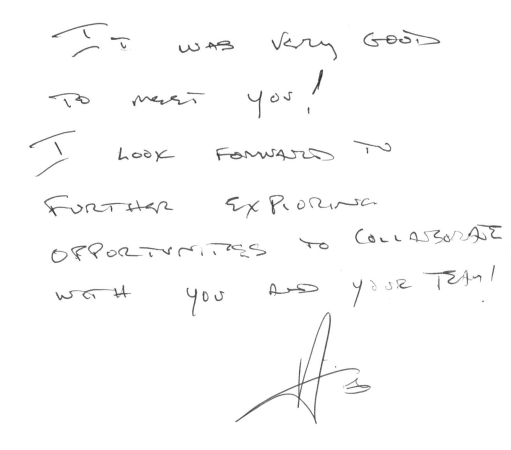

CONCUSSION–OLOGY

Redefining Sports Concussion Management For All Levels

ATHLETES
PARENTS
COACHES
ATHLETIC TRAINERS
LEAGUE OFFICIALS
REFEREES
MEDICAL PROFESSIONALS

HARRY KERASIDIS, M.D.

authorHOUSE®

AuthorHouse™
1663 Liberty Drive
Bloomington, IN 47403
www.authorhouse.com
Phone: 1 (800) 839-8640

Published by AuthorHouse   09/09/2015

ISBN: 978-1-5049-2515-0 (sc)
ISBN: 978-1-5049-2516-7 (e)

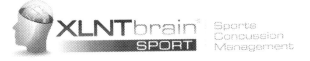

137 National Plaza, Suite 300, National Harbor MD 20745
(855) 333-9568, info@xlntbrain.com
www.xlntbrain.com

"*That Dr. Kerasidis is as open-minded and forward-thinking as he is intellectually brilliant, speaks to the genius of his work in the medical field. I can attest to this as a person who crossed his path while seeking answers on her own journey to better brain health. This book is a reflection of that genius: straightforward, smart and leading-edge.*"

— Erin Sharoni
National TV Sports Personality, CBS Sports

"*Dr. Kerasidis explains the brain in user-friendly terms, including how it functions normally and how it responds in concussion (mild traumatic brain injury, TBI). He recognizes the same critically important research studies as I do in my papers on the neuroimaging and treatment of TBI. He emphasizes the long-lasting changes from mild TBI which can persist for a lifetime. This book offers a window into the sports culture that surrounds concussion and is a clear call to action for players, parents, coaches, and loved ones.*"

— Theodore Henderson, MD, PhD
Child, Adolescent, and General Psychiatry

"*As an athletic trainer I work with concussions every day. Therefore I need to be able to recognize, diagnose, and manage concussions as if it were a textbook lateral ankle sprain. Dr. Kerasidis expertise in concussions and concussion management has taught me what I need to know and helped me become a better athletic trainer. A concussion or mild traumatic brain injury can be a very scary and devastating injury. However with his guidance and expertise I have been able to treat people with the best possible care and outcome. He truly is an expert in the field of concussions and sports and has helped me develop and implement a first class concussion management program.*"

— Stephanie Guzzo
Assistant Athletic Trainer, St. Mary's College of Maryland

"Cognitive neurologist Harry Kerasidis has presented a full, all inclusive approach to the management of sports related concussions, as well a program for brain health, in his book "Concussionology: Redefining Sports Concussion Management For All Levels." Dr. Kerasidis, also called the Brain Doctor, a well deserved title for the time and efforts he has put forth in developing his concussion management programs, leads us through the basics of brain anatomy and function and what happens when a "brain sprain" occurs. Citing scientific studies, Dr. Kerasidis presents data for the management of concussions, debunking some of the myths that have accumulated over the past fifty years. He has suggested some basics ideas on the handling of concussions, as well as improving the concussed athlete's chances for returning to participation in sports, as well as everyday life, with a well functioning brain. While Dr. Kerasidis program refers to sports concussions, brain trauma and cognitive impairment occurs in non-athletes as well, and his program for rehabilitation and recovery can be applied to these individuals. His book cites many references and websites for the reader to examine each topic and question in depth. This book will provide experts as well as budding "concussionologists" with a wealth of material."

— Dr. Alan Ashare, Board member, USA Hockey

Dr. Alan Ashare has been an advocate for safety in sports for over three decades. Starting the "Head Up, Don't Duck" Program in ice hockey in 1995 to decrease the risk for catastrophic paralyzingly neck injuries. He serves on the Board of Directors of USA Hockey and is active in sports medicine committees for Massachusetts high schools and the Massachusetts Medical Society. He is active in helping to develop standards for sports safety equipment with the American Society for Testing and Materials, and has organized multiple ASTM international conferences on sports safety. He is a coauthor with Bill and Katharine White of the book "Winning the War Against Concussions in Youth Sports."

CONTENTS

CHAPTER 1

INTRODUCTION

The Emerging Field of Sports and Medicine

Athletes, young and old, are struggling with concussions and the effects of this mild traumatic brain injury, often whether they realize it or not. The modern sports culture is colliding with neurological intelligence, forcing athletes to decide between getting more "game-time" or preserving a healthy brain.

Today's athletes must become aware of concussions and the blank stares, confusion, memory loss, and other symptoms that can accompany the brain injury, which I will explain in this book. But there's more to concussions than just knowing the symptoms because each concussion can lead to significant problems in the future. Yet the sports culture that breeds "toughness," hoping for scholarships, and professional big-time income, may be pulling the wrong end of the tug-of-war. In the end, the wealth that lures many young athletes is not worth the cognitive and emotional consequences that could impede a happy, healthy life.

The athletes aren't alone. Parents, coaches, athletic trainers, league officials, and virtually everybody else involved with supporting athletic development are grasping for answers too. Concussions are in the limelight now, and virtually all sports levels and individuals are looking to understand what can be done to assure athletes avoid the dangerous risk of short- and long-term cognitive and emotional impairment resulting from concussion injuries.

Concussion incidence rates are much higher than most realize. Many athletes in contact sports experience a concussion more often than they actually report. The Center for Disease Control (CDC) estimate more than 3 million concussions occur every year in the United States. If we calculate all the hits in practice—hits off the field, jarring falls, whiplash effects from driving accidents, even falls as a child—the incidence rates of concussions far exceed what we can estimate.

The growing number of lawsuits by former players in the National Football League (NFL) and National Hockey League (NHL) have brought concussions and brain trauma to the spotlight in recent years. The trickle down has affected the National Collegiate Athletic Association (NCAA), and inevitably will reach the high school and youth league levels. Similar to the domino effect, a trail of repercussions has followed including: daily news reports about concussions; states establishing concussion education laws; documentaries have been filmed; and, the scientific community has a new frontier to discover. This has caused a rapid convergence of consensus statements and guidelines regarding the management of sport-related concussions to be written, forcing the sports world to reexamine their knowledge about the brain and how to protect it.

Still, questions remain about how the sports world will effectively manage concussions moving into the future, and equally important how it will begin to change its culture.

The cultural change may be the most difficult. For example, I would love to say that gone are the days that we call a concussion a "ding" or "getting your bell rung." Respected organizations such as the National Athletic Trainers Association (NATA) have put forth guidelines calling for an end to references like these because they minimize the serious nature of concussion injury. Still, these references still permeate throughout our society. Dizzy athletes are told to "walk it off" by their coaches. Athletes fail to report their symptoms for fear that they will not be allowed to play. Team doctors push pills to mask the symptoms in professional athletes. In the end, it is the athlete's brain that suffers from mismanagement of the concussion injury due to this minimization. Risks of prolonged symptoms, long-term impairments of memory and thinking, emotional consequences, and early dementia seem to be blocked out of the picture. There must be a cultural shift in the sports world to prioritize brain health over gameplay in order to correct this phenomenon.

Unfortunately, parents and coaches aren't typically well versed in brain matters. The sports therapy and athletic trainer industries have been strapped with outdated learning, inconvenient tools and techniques.

The phrase "sports concussion management" is still a relatively new concept that can bring a number of individuals to the table for a neurological decision. For the purpose of this book, let's define sports concussion management as: *A system to prevent, detect and protect athletes from concussion injury, including protocols for education, baseline testing, sideline assessments, post-injury care and return-to-play decisions.*

This leaves most sports teams with the task of piecing together various materials, tests, and tools to create protocols that helps prevent, detect, and protect athletes from significant brain damage. The heightened awareness of the effects of concussions has created a need for a single reliable and practical source of information that provides expert guidance.

That's why it's time for "Concussionology," as I hope to define best practices in sports concussion management and this emerging new field of sports and medicine.

As a cognitive neurologist, I've specialized in concussions, and particularly the behavioral alterations associated with brain trauma. After nearly 25 years studying the brain and treating hundreds, perhaps thousands, of concussions, I've seen a gap between what happens on and off the field, and what doctors and scientists really know about concussions. So, I wrote this book to help bridge the gap.

My conclusion is that the sports world is starving to benefit from neurology and new technology to create a seamless, thorough, and practical sports-concussion-management solution that can be applied in all sports and at all levels. I've organized my protocol with the following "Four Rs:"

Recognize — Take advantage of desktop and mobile platforms to deliver proper awareness of: the potential ravages of concussions; state laws compliance to concussion prevention recommendations; and educational information that the athlete and all those people that surround the athlete need to be able to detect the presence, severity, and recovery of concussion-related symptoms. This includes preseason baseline testing that measure the full spectrum of cognitive and emotional performance tasks prior to possible seasonal injuries, in an effort to detect subtle effects of brain trauma.

Report — Encourage athletes to report their injury or when they observe an injured teammate, and develop a culture that prioritizes brain health over gameplay. This culture would help protect athletes from dangers associated with playing with a concussion. Also be sure to gather, document and report important data regarding the athlete's condition, utilizing a sideline assessment — preferably on a mobile platform. This informs all the individuals, and medical professionals responsible for the health of the athlete, with data within minutes of the injury occurring.

Recover — Guide the athlete and training staff through a progressive exertion protocol that helps determine when the athlete can be cleared for "return to gameplay," as well as "return to learn" for all academic activities. Provide a mobile tool that helps with "symptom tracking" throughout the process.

Responsibility — It takes a "team effort" to apply concussion management. The team includes athletes, parents, coach, training staff, medical professionals, referees, and league officials. The health of the athlete's short- and long-term future should weigh heavier on brain health than the desire to have the athlete to return to the field.

With the connectivity of the Internet, mobile applications, and advances in information technology, an end-to-end approach is now available to relieve the growing concern of brain health for athletes. When referring to an "end-to-end" solution, I'm referring to a program that can be implemented for all sports and all levels from the beginning of the season to the return of an athlete to normal activity and gameplay. Here are some examples of technological advances that could be applied to a clinical-caliber concussion management program:

- Internet-based computer technology offers a centralized method of accomplishing each of the steps in the process, and the ability to integrate everything into a single source, which has never been done before.
- Online video training provides improved efficiency in educating proper concussion awareness for athletes, parents, coaches, and

educators to optimize prevention, recognize the presence of concussion-related symptoms, and encourage a cultural shift towards prioritizing brain health over gameplay.

- Smartphone technology is now at a level of sophistication to integrate assessment tools to assist responsible adults at the sidelines to document potential concussion incidents. This technology also allows injured players a convenient method of documenting concussion-related symptoms during the post concussion recovery phase.
- The immediate connectivity of the Internet and email allows for instant alerts of potential concussion events to all key individuals involved in athlete's care. Athletic trainers and other healthcare providers can track injured athletes' recovery progress in real-time, making post concussion management as efficient as possible. If all the concussion management elements were integrated into one platform, then reporting becomes simplified and equips all the parties involved with access to the data. For example, school administrators can instantly access data related to athletes' and parents' completion of state mandated preseason activities, and policies and procedures.
- A fully integrated computer-based system also allows for the objectivity and transparency needed to manage concussions properly under the watchful eyes of league officials and union administrators.

Research applications using a comprehensive, fully integrated, computerized concussion management system abound. Possible applications include: evaluation of potential bio-markers for the vulnerability of concussion; the development of delayed effects of multiple brain trauma; clinical correlation of concussion incidence; severity to bio-mechanical measures such as accelerometer technology. I also think my concussion management platform could help us understand the effects of therapeutic interventions on recovery time and cognitive performance.

Retired athletes can also reap the benefits of a fully-integrated, computer-based system. A digital "concussion tracker" can follow an athlete through all levels of play through a lifetime, from youth levels to high school, collegiate, professional, and even through retirement. Players who are cognitively asymptomatic can document their cognitive performance and experience of symptoms related to brain function online as part of a surveillance program meant for early detection and treatment of delayed effects of multiple brain trauma.

A complete sports concussion management program, as described here, gives the sports world a chance to have a "virtual neurologist" on its team, ultimately preserving the athletes' health and optimizing their game performance.

Utilizing technology, my own neurology expertise, and experience, I've created a sports concussion management program that rivals the NFL's, and is now being adopted by thousands of people on the youth, high school, and collegiate levels. It includes a fully-integrated, comprehensive, clinical-caliber concussion management system, which can be implemented easily for all sports and levels. I've written this book to share the principles of my program, while giving readers a healthy dose of understanding the concussion injury and related repercussions.

In **Concussionology: Redefining Sports Concussion Management**, I'll give you a crash course about the neurology of the brain and behavior, deconstruct concussions, and discuss the repercussions of concussions on cognitive and emotional behaviors. This book will also layout a sports concussion management game-plan that benefits from technological advances to simplify and enhance concussion management for anyone, any sport of any level. The overall goal is to protect athletes from brain damage caused from trauma, while helping them enjoy the many lessons and experiences enjoyed from playing in the games themselves. Concussions don't have to kill contact sports. We just need greater awareness, proper tools and shift the culture to put brain health above wins and losses.

## CHAPTER 2

HARRY'S STORY

The Start of Concussionology Begins with My Own Concussion

It was late October, my freshman year of college, at George Washington University and I was home for my local high school's Homecoming weekend. It was a beautiful Sunday afternoon, not that I remember much more than that.

A bunch of guys from my neighborhood decided to get together for a friendly game of tackle football—without pads or helmets—at the field of the elementary school nearby. I drove my car, an aging Mercury Capri, whose valves had recently gone bad, requiring an overhaul earlier in the week. I arrived, and we lined up five-on-five that afternoon, with girlfriends and friends sitting on a small hill at one end of the field like bleachers in a stadium.

My team kicked off. I raced down the field, carrying the inertia of a 6'1," 170-pound young man running at full speed to stop the receiver, Hank, a tall lanky guy. He *tried* to evade my tackle unsuccessfully. I led with my head colliding with his bony hip. That's where my memory for the events that followed become sketchy.

My best friend, and girl-next-door, Ellen filled in the blanks for me. Apparently, I didn't get up and huddle after the play as I normally would. Instead, I sat on the field, rubbing my head on both sides with my hands in a twisting motion. My buddies had not noticed at first, because Hank was howling and running around yelling, "Ouch! My hip!" When they noticed me, my friends, Johnny and Andy came over to see if I was okay. I couldn't really tell them, all I could do was just look at them. So Johnny suggested that I sit the next play out. I went up to the hill and sat by Ellen.

"Are you alright?" she asked.

"Yeah, I think I hit my head. I'm just going to sit the next play out," I said.

Questions That Led to More Questions

"What was the play that I got hit on?" I asked. She told me that it was the kickoff play and what happened.

"Okay, I guess I will just sit out this next play."

We sat and watched as the game continued. A few minutes later, I asked her what happened to me.

"What was the play that I got hit on?" And she described it all over again.

"Oh," I said, not talking much, just sitting and watching. A few more minutes went by and I asked her again, "What was the play that I got hit on?"

At this point, Ellen was getting concerned. She called Andy over, telling him, "Harry is confused."

Andy started asking me questions. "Do you remember getting your car fixed earlier this week?" I stared blankly back at him.

"No, I haven't fixed it yet, I have to save up some money."

He and Ellen did not know what to do with such a response since I was so happy when I finally got my car back from the shop.

"Harry, you picked your car up last Wednesday. Look you drove it here!" Ellen said.

I looked up at the parking lot and saw my car there. "No, I'm sure it's not fixed yet," I said, not even processing the fact that I wouldn't have driven it if it had not been repaired.

After arguing the matter and my personal finances with them for a few minutes, I walked up the hill, popped the hood, and started revving the engine. I was so impaired that I could not determine that, in fact, it was running just fine, without the nasty noises an engine with bad valves makes.

Andy and Ellen followed me up. "See? It's running great!" Andy said.

"I can't tell," I said resolutely.

We went back and sat down on the grass. "Do you remember taking Shelley to the homecoming dance last night?" they asked.

"No, why would I do that?" I replied.

Shelley was a very nice girl that lived in my neighborhood, but she was not my girlfriend. They reminded me that she had an extra ticket, and that she asked me to take her, which was great because it gave me the opportunity to get together with her and all of my friends from the neighborhood. I could not recall any of the events from the night before.

Once again, I asked Ellen what happened to me, and why my head was hurting. "What was the play that I got hit on?"

Ellen suggested that maybe I should go home. I agreed. I insisted on driving, she decided to accompany me. The drive was not far and we made it back uneventfully.

Intervention Arrives

Ellen and I entered the house and my mother was on the second floor greeting us from the top of the stairs. "Hi, how are you?" I just stared back, like a deer in the headlights. My mother thought I had taken drugs. Ellen quickly explained that I had hit my head and was confused. Seeing my vacant stare and confused state my mother decided to drive me to the emergency room.

As my mom drove she asked me questions like what's our phone number and our address, which I knew. I even could tell her when to make the correct turns to go to the hospital. In spite of passing those basic cognitive questions, mom said I was eerily quiet and not talkative.

We made it to the hospital and checked in to the ER. "Why am I here?" I asked my mother, and she told me. "How did we get here?" I asked.

I was evaluated by the ER doctor who ordered a CT scan. As I was wheeled out of the CT scanner suite, my mother asked me "What did you do in there?"

"In where?" I replied.

"In that room, that you just came out," she said.

"I haven't been in there," I replied. To this day, I still don't know what it is like to lay in a CT scanner.

The Mysterious, Lucky Rabbit Foot

By this time, my father had come, with my little sister. The previous weekend, I had been at the beach in Ocean City, Maryland and I had won a "lucky rabbit's foot" key chain at one of the boardwalk games and given it to my sister. She was wearing it on a belt loop on her jeans that day.

"Hey, Marsha, that's a cool rabbit's foot, where did you get it?" She was quite surprised at the question, and told me that I had given it to her. In the next couple of hours, I had asked her the same question so many times that she decided to hide the rabbit's foot in her pocket just so I wouldn't ask any more.

The doctor told my parents that my CT scan was normal, but because my confusion and amnesia were persistent, they were going to admit me to the hospital for observation overnight.

Out of sheer coincidence, I was put in a double room with a guy I had gone to high school with. "Danah! How are you doing! Long time no see! What are you doing here?"

He explained that he was admitted for a hip operation that he was going to have the next day. The nurses came in and drew the curtain between us to do the intake evaluation. Once they were done, they pulled the curtain back and I saw Danah again.

"Danah! How are you doing! Long time no see! What are you doing here?"

He looked at my mother and said, "Harry is really messed up isn't he?"

After I asked the same questions to Danah two or three more times, which was each time the curtain between us was drawn and then pulled back, the nurses decided to move me to a private room to give Danah some rest.

The next day, I was pretty much back to normal. I was discharged and went home to rest before going back to my college classes. The whole event made for good stories, and to this day the question, "Where did you get that rabbit's foot?" has been a running joke in my family.

I was perplexed after that event, however. How was it that I could behave and interact relatively normal, even drive and give directions, and have absolutely no memory of those events? It was a lost weekend for me. I could not even verify my own existence during that time, and yet I seemed to be functioning.

These questions profoundly influenced me and compelled me to study the brain and ultimately become a neurologist. Later, I learned that I had classic signs of injury to the temporal lobes. The temporal lobes support short-term memory. I was exhibiting textbook signs of acute concussion injury including *retrograde amnesia* (loss of memory for events that happened before the injury, like taking Shelley to the homecoming dance) and *anterograde amnesia* (loss of memory for events that took place after the injury, like being in the CT scanner). Although less pronounced, I also experienced concussion-related headaches and fatigue.

Moving Forward

After reading this book, you will have a better grasp of the medical terminology dealing with the brain and hopefully gain a new level of respect for concussions. Sometimes, I refer to a concussion as if it's a "brain sprain." Please note that I use terms like "brain sprain" and "brain drain" not to minimize the seriousness of the concussion injury, but rather to help with providing the reader terms easier to relate to and understand. One thing I've learned in my years treating concussions is that no two concussions are alike and each presents its own unique constellation of symptoms.

## CHAPTER 3

BRAIN BRIEFING

WARNING: Contents Are Fragile

The brain is beautiful—the new frontier of science, but the brain is also vulnerable. It's fragile, gel-like consistency floats unattached inside the skull. When force is applied, which occurs many times in sports collisions, the brain sloshes from side to side and end to end, almost like scrambling the yolk of an egg as it floats inside without breaking its shell.

The symptoms of concussions and undiagnosed brain injuries can be seen immediately or can take several hours or even days for symptoms to materialize. But their effects can be life-altering. It's a mystery that science and the sports world are unraveling. The sports world has to unravel this mystery because the quality of lives and futures are at stake, which until recently, had not been as important as wins and losses.

For example, the *Wall Street Journal* reported on the front page in 2008 that undiagnosed brain injuries are a major cause of:

- Homelessness
- Psychiatric illness
- Depression and anxiety
- Alcoholism and drug abuse
- Suicide
- Learning problems

To better understand concussions, first we need a better understanding of the brain itself. It's a wonderfully complex organ, and "command central" literally responsible for regulating or executing every move we make, every word we say, every emotion we feel, and every thought we think. The healthy brain is precious to life. Therefore, preserving its health is the key to a long life, full of memories, special moments, and success.

In this chapter, I want to instill in you a healthy respect for the brain and its functions. You don't have to be a neurologist to manage concussions, but I believe the more you understand the brain, the more you will understand the implications of suffering brain trauma and the potential for short- and long-term consequences.

Brain health is so critical to proper life functioning that maybe helmets should include a label, "WARNING: Contents Are Fragile."

Brain Matters

The consistency of the brain is somewhere between slightly-set gelatin and peanut butter—almost like impressionable memory-foam pillows.

I think people underestimate how powerful, yet vulnerable the brain is. Since we don't see the brain, we take it for granted. Unlike injuries you can see, like scrapes, cuts, sprains, bruise, or breaks, it's easy to overlook the role the brain plays, particularly when it experiences trauma.

Despite being encased within a stone-like skull, the brain can be easily affected by outside trauma. Its soft texture is impressionable, like a banana. So when the brain bounces inside the skull, it doesn't immediately spring back into shape. The brain is in continual use, carrying out numerous voluntary and involuntary functions every second, so when it experiences trauma—like a hard fall or direct hit to the head—normal functioning can be interrupted momentarily or for longer periods of time.

Since we can't see the brain, unless we use a form of scanning (Chapter 5), we must assess potential brain damage from a variety of visible or felt symptoms and from measuring brain performance.

Clearly, the brain matters. It's fascinating to me how the body and brain automatically regulate so many functions simultaneously and involuntarily. The brain directs our body to digest food we eat, signals the heart when and how to react, administers healing when it perceives trouble, including many other functions. When the brain experiences a form of trauma, whether physical, mental, or emotional, it has the power to begin a self-healing process.

It's important to note that our conscious, or voluntary behaviors can influence the healing process as well. For example, the kind of food we eat either helps or hurts our brain. Getting enough sleep and drinking enough water influences the brain. Toxic chemicals from tobacco smoke, drug use, alcohol, and even fumes from paint or fumes from hair and nail salons can drastically reduce the brain's effectiveness.

When the brain is traumatized, many of its functions can be compromised, as you will see in Chapter 6.

Brain Basics

By learning the fundamental principles of brain structure and function, you will better understand the sensitive relationship between the brain and its internal and external environments. We can alter the function of the brain either positively or negatively, and knowing the basics, we can be better prepared to prevent or detect neurological trauma.

- First, the brain is not a uniform mass of tissue. It's made of several sections, responsible for various functions. The brain is also composed of billions of specialized cells called neurons and glia.
- The brain floats within fluid inside the skull that has ridges and shelf-like areas, which is why it is vulnerable to jarring hits or whiplash-type action.
- The brain requires significant blood flow and oxygen to operate. The brain makes up about 2 percent of our body weight, but consumes 20 percent of the oxygen we breathe and 20 percent of the energy we consume.
- This enormous consumption of oxygen and energy fuels billions of chemical reactions in the brain every second. This is perhaps one of the most motivating reasons to provide the right kind of fuel for the brain by consuming a healthy diet and performing regular exercise.

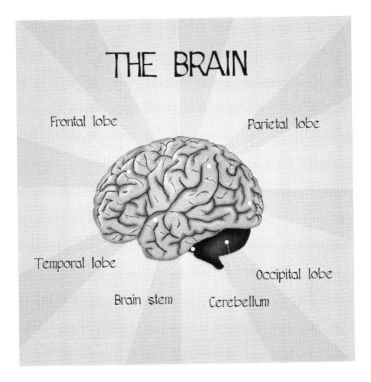

Brain Anatomy

Don't let the word "anatomy" intimidate you. As you learn about the brain, you will discover many scientific terms, but I tried not to overload this material with "unnecessary" neurological terms. Let me assure you, the word anatomy is not one of those unnecessary terms. Simply put, anatomy is the understanding of the physical parts of the brain and their related functions. Since I believe "Concussionology" is becoming a new field in sports and science, you need to know basic anatomy to be able to see how concussions can affect virtually every system in the brain and body.

Regions

The brain is organized into three main sections: the cerebrum, cerebellum, and the brainstem, which are then divided into more specific areas. Trauma received in any of the three main sections tends to cause problems associated with that area's functions. Any sudden movement with force can result in the brain sliding back and forth, which can cause temporary and permanent cognitive damage. "Cognitive" refers to conscious mental activities such as thinking, reasoning, understanding, learning, memory, language, coordination, and emotion.

The most vulnerable areas of the brain are the frontal and temporal sides (lobes) due to their anatomy and proximity to the skull.

Frontal: Responsible for executive functioning, forethought, planning, organizing, complex thinking, focus and concentration, emotional self-regulation.

Temporal: Responsible for auditory processing, short-term memory, and mood regulation.

Below is a general overview of the sections of the brain and their associated behaviors, which can be affected by concussions and more severe brain trauma.

Cerebrum

The cerebrum or the "forebrain" is the largest section of the brain and is divided into left and right regions called hemispheres.

Prefrontal Cortex (PFC): The PFC is located in the front third of the brain—in the forehead above the eyes where most hits to the head are sustained in football. The PFC is particularly noteworthy because its role is to supervise the rest of your brain and body. It's like your own personal CEO for life, serving to make decisions, pay attention, make judgments, plan, control impulses, know when to follow-through, and when to empathize. Conversely, damage to the PFC can result in poor decision-making, impulsivity, short attention span, lack of goal setting, and procrastination.

Anterior Cingulate Gyrus (ACG): Running lengthwise under the PFC, the ACG regulates our ability to shift attention when needed, adapt to change, and be flexible in thought and reasoning. When this area of the brain is not working properly, people can get stuck on negative thoughts or actions, become overly worrisome, hold grudges, and be oppositional or argumentative. Another word for these related behaviors is "compulsive." For example, "compulsive gambling" is when a person can't quit even when they realize it is compromising their livelihood. This shows a traumatized ACG.

Temporal Lobes: Located on the left and right side, underneath the temples, and behind your eyes, the **temporal lobes** are involved in auditory processing, language, short-term memory, mood, and temper stability. They also help interpret and name what things are. These lobes often experience trauma from jarring hits from contact and collision sports that can lead to problems with memory, mood, and temper.

Parietal Lobes: Located in the back, top part of the brain, the parietal lobes are involved with sensory processing, spatial relations, and direction sense. Typically, Alzheimer's disease will impact this area, giving people with this condition a hard time with finding their way resulting in them getting lost. Other problems with parietal lobes can lead to inaccurate interpretations of body perception.

Occipital Lobes: The occipital lobes, located in the back of the brain, are involved with vision and visual processing. Information taken through the eyes are sorted out in the occipital lobes and dispersed to the various regions of the brain for action.

Limbic System (LS): Arching deep inside the brain, from the frontal lobes through the parietal lobes to the temporal lobes, the LS helps set your emotional tone, either positive and hopeful or negative and desperate. Problems with the LS have been linked to low motivation, poor self-esteem, feelings of depression, helplessness, and hopelessness.

Cerebellum

The "hindbrain" is located in the back area toward the base of the skull. Working in tandem with the PFC, the cerebellum is the "coordinator," involved with voluntary physical (motor) movements, posture, balance, coordination, as well as processing speed. This coordination is also linked to enable the PFC's role of helping with judgment and impulse control. Trouble with the cerebellum leads to coordination problems, and ability to learn.

Brainstem

The brainstem is the portion of the brain that is directly connected to the spinal cord at the base of the brain.

The brainstem relays signals from the brain throughout the body, controlling and regulating vital body functions including respiration, heart rate, and blood pressure. The brainstem also contains the relay centers for the control of information to and from various parts of the head including the coordination of eye movements, facial movement and sensation, hearing, balance, and control of the mouth and tongue

The brain processes information by splitting a single behavior into components. For example, when we take a bite of food, there is *sensory* information (this is an apple), *voluntary motor* information (lift piece to mouth, chew), and *involuntary motor* information (salivate) for the brain to process. The different components are split, sent to the appropriate regions of the brain, and then processed accordingly.

If there is trauma experienced in any of these processes, the brain's ability to process the appropriate behavior can be affected.

Input and Output

The brain is continuously processing sensory-input signals received from the eyes, ears, nose, mouth, and skin. In addition to the traditional five senses, scientists now recognize other kinds of sensory inputs, including pain, pressure, temperature, joint position, and movement. The brain then organizes and directs appropriate responses (motor output), voluntary—conscious decisions, or involuntary—in which the brain decides for us. This interaction between input and output is supervised by the Central

Nervous System (CNS) and executed by the Peripheral Nervous System (PNS).

Central Nervous System

The CNS is like a computer's central processing unit (CPU) for the body. Coordinating the brain and body, the CNS receives sensory inputs from the body, and Peripheral Nervous System, to initiate appropriate action—or motor outputs (coordinated mechanical responses). Working through the spinal cord, the CNS determines what input needs to be filtered through the brain and where it needs to be sent throughout the body—its muscles and glands. Interestingly enough, at least to me, not all motor responses require conscious brain processing. The CNS is able to direct certain action immediately if needed, as in a knee-jerk reflex.

More complex motor actions, whether voluntary or some involuntary, require more brain involvement. The brain is the "director" of information throughout the body, devoting most of its volume and computational power to processing various sensory inputs to determine and initiate appropriate and coordinated motor output.

Peripheral Nervous System

The PNS is composed of nerve tissue outside the brain and spinal cord, serving to deliver the information between the body and CNS for the brain to process. It carries messages from the body's sensory organs and voluntary muscles, giving us the ability to detect changes in the environment around us and deliver that information to the CNS for direction on what actions to perform. Additionally, the PNS carries messages between the CNS and our internal organs, regulating automatic tasks such as breathing and digesting—called the autonomic nervous system.

Brain Talk

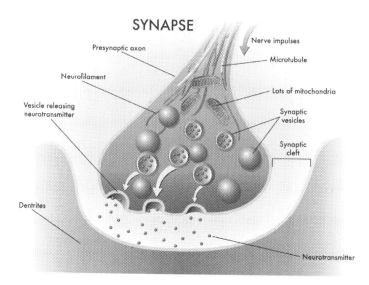

SYNAPSE

Presynaptic axon

Neurofilament

Vesicle releasing neurotransmitter

Dentrites

Nerve impulses

Microtubule

Lots of mitochondria

Synaptic vesicles

Synaptic cleft

Neurotransmitter

The brain uses neurons to communicate to itself. Neurons are the functional cells that receive and transmit information to other neurons and cells. This transmission of information enables us to react to changes in our internal and external environments.

Neurons send and receive messages through a two-part process called *neural signaling.* Neural signaling begins with an electrical impulse generated when a stimulus (such as sensory input) and causes a rapid change in electrical charge in one part of a neuron's membrane. This electrical impulse is one unit of neural information. An electrical impulse flowing along the length of a neuron is called a nerve impulse. The ability to generate this electrical impulse depends on the neuron's ability to maintain a very precise balance and equilibrium of salts such as potassium and sodium, inside and outside the cell membrane. Much of the energy requirements of the neuron are devoted to maintaining this equilibrium.

For that impulse to leap the synapse (gap between cells, neurons) to another cell and create the desired communication, the neuron releases chemical messenger molecules known as *neurotransmitters.*

Brain Gain

The brain develops rapidly throughout pregnancy and early childhood. Neurons are making billions of connections during the first few years of a human's life. The brain continues developing until the age of 25 years for most. Scientific investigations have demonstrated that even the adult brain generates new neurons within a region important for learning and memory. The brain's ability to change and reorganize in response to some input is known as *plasticity*.

Learning is a form of plasticity, since it leads to structural changes in the brain. While brain plasticity can be gained, it can also be drained. Brain drain, as we will get into in Chapters 5 and 6, is considered to be degenerative but also highly dependent on the health of the brain. The health of the brain is largely dependent on lifestyle factors, brain injuries, and brain-related training.

All this brain anatomy, brain talk, and brain gain discussions are meant to establish a foundation of understanding of the brain and resulting effects of a concussion. When the brain is traumatized, there can be lapses within the typical brain function, which is revealed through symptoms. These lapses can lead to future cognitive and emotional impairment.

Now, let's open the Concussionology discussion further, and learn about the brain injury called concussion.

CHAPTER 4

DEFINING "BRAIN SPRAIN"

The Ultimate One-Hit Wonder

Little did I know an afternoon playing tackle football among friends could change my life forever, and for the better. After that fateful tackle introduced my head to my friend's hip rather forcefully, it caused a series of repercussions, still being felt today. It was the ultimate one-hit wonder that gave me temporary memory loss, established my career destiny, and led me to helping many, many people understand concussions.

Looking back, I feel lucky. Although my concussion served as a wake-up call, it healed without further incident and I was able to continue my education, start a family and build a career. Unfortunately, concussions don't always end so well for others. Concussions can end careers, cause life-long headaches, memory loss, emotional disturbances and many other forms cognitive impairment (*see* Chapters 5, 6).

Let's get more familiar with the brain injury known as a concussion, which often gets minimized with terms like getting your "bell rung," "clocked," or a "ding." I've termed it a "brain sprain," to help with associating the injury with something more familiar. However, please do not interpret "brain sprain" as a trivial injury. A concussion is like a "sprain" because of associated tissue injury. Rest is required for recovery and on occasion rest can be prolonged and have long-term consequences if not treated properly. The key difference between an "ankle sprain" and "brain sprain" are the more dire repercussions associated with a brain sprain affecting cognitive, emotional, and behavioral functions. These impairments can drastically alter the course of life.

Incidence Rates in Sports

Almost every sport puts players at risk of a concussion. While collision sports are obviously the riskiest, a jarring fall or untimely hit to the head occur more often than you think. Even if you don't play a sport, concussions can occur in every day life, at any age, and with varying levels of severity.

Emergency rooms across the nation are reporting increased incidents in sports-related concussions. In my practice, I've seen a dramatic increase in the number of patients reporting sports-related concussions in the last 10 years. I believe this is due partly to increased awareness, and other factors like bigger, faster, and more aggressive athletes, as well as the increased participation of women in sports.

Unfortunately, there's really no way of accurately tracking every concussion because most athletes don't want to pull themselves out of the game or practice. Various studies have attempted to measure the number of concussions, and which sport is the biggest culprit. While I appreciate good science, there is a wide range of data making it difficult to accurately estimate. For our purposes, let's go with the following numbers to give you an idea of concussion prevalence in the United States, and which sports have the highest incidence rates.

- An estimated 300,000 sports-related concussions are recorded at emergency rooms every year, accounting for nearly 10 percent of all high school sports injuries, and 20 percent of all football injuries.
- The Center for Disease Control estimates as many as 3.8 million sports and recreational-activity related concussions occur each year in the United States alone. However, as many as 90% of concussions go unreported.

Concussions occur in all sports with the highest incidence in football, hockey, rugby, soccer, basketball, wrestling, and lacrosse. Even cheerleading accidents report high in concussion incidence. In fact, one study showed

10 percent of all high school sports concussions came from wrestling and cheerleading.

According to *Epidemiology of Concussions Among United States High School Athletes in 20 Sports*,[1] the study ranked the majority of concussions occur from these sports:

1. Football (47.1%)
2. Girls' soccer (8.2%)
3. Boys' wrestling (5.8%)
4. Girls' basketball (5.5%)

Other findings from the same study showed, football had the highest concussion rate (6.4), followed by boys' ice hockey (5.4), and boys' lacrosse (4.0). Concussions represented a greater proportion of total injuries among boys' ice hockey (22.2%) than all other sports studied (13.0%) (injury proportion ratio).

Breaking down football in further detail:

- About 40% of concussions occur when tackling, 25% when being tackled.
- 30% occur in linebackers and running backs.
- Over 60% occur from helmet-to-helmet contact.

A growing concern is concussions in high school girls' soccer. Studies show girls are reporting nearly twice as many concussions as boys. Not only that, the number of girls suffering concussions in soccer accounts for the second largest amount of all concussions reported by young athletes. This information is according to the Center for Injury Research and Policy in Columbus, Ohio.

---

[1] Center for Injury Research and Policy, The Research Institute at Nationwide Children's Hospital. *Epidemiology of Concussions Among United States High School Athletes in 20 Sports* (Columbus, OH 43205, USA) http://www.ncbi.nlm. nih.gov/pubmed/22287642.

Concussion Definition

So what is a concussion? Does every hit to the head cause one? How severe is a concussion? Does a loss of consciousness qualify as a concussion? Let's begin to answer these foundational questions.

Concussion Is a Brain Injury

Think of a bruised banana—in simple terms, that's what a concussion is like. The banana's interior can suffer damage when enough force is felt by the exterior.

As mentioned above, you may *think of a concussion like a brain sprain*, because it's usually disabling, but typically a person can recover from the disability in time and with a lot of rest. Like an ankle sprain, a concussion has temporary consequences, and if not healed properly, can result in residual and degenerative difficulties. You may be able to continue playing on an ankle sprain and brain sprain, but if you do the risk of greater injury increases. As with ankle sprains, the severity is often minimized and that's something you don't want to do with the brain.

Here are some other more "official" concussion definitions:

> *Concussion is recognized as a clinical syndrome of biomechanically-induced alteration of brain function, typically affecting memory and orientation, which may involve loss of consciousness (LOC).*

> — American Academy of Neurology, 2013

A concussion is an injury to the brain that results in temporary loss of normal brain function. A blow to the head usually causes it. Cuts or bruises may be present on the head or face, but in many cases, there are no signs of trauma. Many people assume that concussions involve a loss of consciousness, but that is not true. In most cases, a person with a concussion *never loses consciousness. The formal medical definition of concussion is: <u>a clinical syndrome characterized by immediate and transient alteration in brain function, including alteration of mental status and level of consciousness, resulting from mechanical force or trauma.</u>*

— American Association of
Neurological Surgeons, 2011

A panel discussion regarding the definition of concussion and its separation from mild traumatic brain injury (mTBI) was held. There was acknowledgement by the Concussion in Sport Group (CISG) that although the terms mTBI and concussion are often used interchangeably in the sporting context and particularly in North American literature, others use the term to refer to different injury constructs. Concussion is the historical term representing <u>low-velocity injuries that cause brain "shaking, resulting in clinical symptoms and not necessarily related to a pathological injury.</u> Concussion is a subset of TBI and will be the term used in this document. It was also noted that the term commotio cerebri is often used in Europe and other countries. Minor revisions were made to the definition of concussion, which is defined as follows:

Concussion is a brain injury and is defined as a complex pathophysiological process affecting the brain, induced by biomechanical forces. Several common features that incorporate clinical, pathologic, and biomechanical injury constructs that may be utilized in defining the nature of a concussive head injury include:

- *Concussion may be caused either by a direct blow to the head, face, neck, or elsewhere on the body with an "impulsive" force transmitted to the head.*

- *Concussion typically results in the rapid onset of short-lived impairment of neurological function that resolves spontaneously. In some cases, symptoms and signs may evolve over a number of minutes to hours.*
- *Concussion may result in neuropathological changes, but the acute clinical symptoms largely reflect a functional disturbance rather than a structural injury and, as such, no abnormality is seen on standard structural neuro-imaging studies.*
- *Concussion results in a graded set of clinical symptoms that may or may not involve loss of consciousness. Resolution of the clinical and cognitive symptoms typically follows a sequential course. It is important to note that in some cases symptoms may be prolonged.*

— Consensus statement on concussion in sport: The 4th International Conference on Concussion in Sport held in Zurich, November 2012

Severity

The severity spectrum of brain injuries range from mild to moderate to severe for concussions. Concussion is widely considered as a mild traumatic brain injury. Concussion is an injury that can last hours, days, and weeks or even months, with the persistent symptom complex referred to as Post-Concussion Syndrome or mild traumatic brain injury (mTBI), which will be explained further in Chapters 5 and 6.

Concussion Signs and Symptoms

<u>*The most important factor to know about signs and symptoms of concussions is that they may not materialize until several minutes, hours, or days after the injury occurs.*</u> This makes concussion detection a tricky business, because the athlete may not make the association of delayed symptoms such as

headache with the collision injury and may want to return to practice or the game.

In Chapter 8, I'll lay out a comprehensive protocol for detection. In the meantime, if an athlete exhibits any of the symptoms below after a hit, pull the athlete aside for a play or two and allow the symptoms to materialize. Despite anyone's desires to get the athlete back in the action, you may be preventing serious risks. After a few minutes of sideline rest, I recommend using my Sideline Assessment Tool and Mobile App to measure the risk and severity of the possible concussion.

Below are explanations of common signs and symptoms. These symptoms result in temporary lapses according to the areas of the brain that have been affected. In the next chapter, we'll review the "Mechanisms of Injury" further.

A variety of signs accompany concussion including somatic symptoms (such as headache and vertigo), impaired cognition (such as difficulty with memory or concentration), emotional extremes (such as worry, mood or anger problems), and abnormal physical signs (such as loss of consciousness, numbness, weakness, and loss of balance).

It's also important to note that any of these symptoms are often present in combination with the others.

Loss of Consciousness: This is the most obvious and scariest sign of a concussion. Only 10 percent of concussions result in loss of consciousness, according to a 2010 *Pediatrics* review article. When a player gets "knocked out" temporarily, the brain continues serving its involuntary functions, but its conscious and voluntary functions discontinue. During this period of time, it's important not to move the individual and allow the brain to "re-boot" for a few seconds. The unconscious athlete should always be assumed to have suffered neck injury with possible spinal instability. Helmets should not be removed and face masks should be cut away should the unconscious athlete require CPR.

Confusion: The most common symptom is temporary confusion, often associated with a "dazed" look or vacant stare. A confused, concussed individual probably won't talk much, because the brain is trying to restore order and understand the circumstances. If the individual does talk, the words may be jumbled, rapid, or generally nonsensical and irrelevant.

Amnesia: This is temporary memory loss that can be divided into two types:

- Retrograde — Forgetting things that happened before the incident.
- Anterograde — Inability to remember facts after the concussion.

Disorientation: Related to spatial relations, a concussion can affect the individual's ability to know where they are, what day it is, and what they were doing at the time of the injury. The athlete may get up and go to the wrong huddle or sideline.

Delayed Verbal/Motor Response: Slow, slurred, or incoherent speech as well as inability to move or walk normally can be associated with concussion.

Inability to Focus: A concussion may be evident if the individual has trouble paying attention and focusing on the conversation or game situation.

Headache: Due to a concussion, headaches that are very similar to migraines complete with nausea, vomiting, and sensory sensitivity may present as a symptom.

Disequilibrium: A problem with balance and feelings of dizziness are common signs.

Visual Disturbances: Vision may become blurred, doubled, or overly sensitive to light.

Nausea/Vomiting: May occur in the absence of headache.

Emotional Liability (mood swings): When hits occur to the sides of the head, or temporal lobes, you may notice anger outbursts, inappropriate laughing, extreme sadness, or overt stubbornness not typical of the individual.

Sleep Disruption: Excessive drowsiness or inability to sleep is usually a delayed symptom of a concussion presumably due to disruption of the sleep pathways rising up through the brainstem and imbalance of the neurotransmitters.

Debunking Common Concussion Myths

Below are the most common myths, and how to steer clear of them.

MYTH: Move the unconscious player immediately off the field for observation.

Wrong: Never move an unconscious individual until a neck or spinal cord injury can be ruled out. Also, do the ABCs; check airway, breathing, and cardiovascular pulse before deciding to if/when/how to move the concussed individual.

MYTH: Need to keep concussed individual awake.

Wrong: In fact, the best and first thing to do is give the concussed brain rest.

MYTH: Concussion symptoms show up immediately.

Wrong: Symptoms don't always occur immediately and can show up hours or even days later.

MYTH: A coach or athlete can decide if they can return to game play based on how hard the hit was or how the athlete says he or she feels.

Wrong: It's impossible to self-diagnose a concussion because judgment can be impaired by whether or not they want to go back in the game. Although the severity of the hit can be a factor, other factors may induce concussions with less violent hits to the head.

MYTH: A well-fitting helmet with the latest technology in protection will prevent concussions.

Wrong: The helmet can prevent injury to the skull, but not the brain. The brain is a soft-tissue, like butter, unattached and encased in fluid. A "whiplash" effect can result in concussion even while wearing a helmet and when no contact is sustained. See "Mechanisms of Injury."

MYTH: Statewide legislation mandating concussion education among contact sports teams is an adequate strategy to preventing, detecting, reporting, and helping concussed athletes return to gameplay safely.

Wrong: Although it's a huge step forward for concussion awareness, most states legislation do not give specifics on how to comply with this law, concussion prevention, concussion detection, and concussion management. Also, education is required, but the state laws loosely monitor and enforce how the education is delivered. Unfortunately, most individuals just need to sign a document—whether or not they've received the training. Additionally, much of the burden is placed on the coaches to comply, and all-involved parties need to be educated.

When a Concussion Is Not a Concussion

It is not uncommon for an athlete to present with signs and symptoms that mimic concussion-related symptoms that are not, in fact, concussion related. Since concussions and their related symptoms are getting so much attention, it's easy to misinterpret other conditions as concussion related. Here are some conditions of symptoms that mimic or can be confused with concussion injury. Remember concussions are a mild brain trauma affecting the physiology of the brain. These conditions below may stand-alone or occur simultaneously with concussion or post-concussion syndrome.

Heat Exhaustion/Dehydration: Many sports begin with practice in the summer months in regions where ambient temperatures on the field may be in the 90s or more. If athletes in these environments do not drink enough water before, during, and after the session then heat exhaustion or dehydration may result. The heat alone may have adverse effects on brain function leading to symptoms such as fainting (loss of consciousness), dizziness, confusion, nausea, vomiting, even convulsions. These symptoms could easily be mistaken for concussion.

Extra Cranial (outside the skull) Soft Tissue Trauma: The head often suffers injury to the tissues outside the skull, particularly in non-helmeted sports. Bruises, lacerations. and other traumatic injury to these tissues are often associated with pain. Attentive care should be taken to address the wound, but be careful not to refer to the pain as a "headache" even though the head may ache.

Occipital Neuritis: A neurological condition often confused with migraines, occipital neuritis involves a pair of nerves at the back of the head below the skull that wrap upwards and around the back of the head to supply sensation to these regions. Injuries that involve "whiplash" movement or rotational forces may stretch and injure these nerves causing inflammation and nerve pain known as *neuralgia*. This pain is usually sharp, stabbing, and radiates up the back of the head or can be dull and aching. Often there is "referred pain" (pain perceived at a location other than the site that received the injury) that is felt behind one or both eyes.

Migraine: Migraine is a common condition occurring equally in about 6 percent of pre-teen boys and girls after the onset of adolescence. The incidence of migraine climbs to about 18 percent in young women while it remains at around 6 percent in men. Migraines run in families. The migraine brain is an irritable brain with unstable physiology and reactivity to many internal and environmental factors, including head trauma. There is significant evidence that having a personal or family history of migraine make one more vulnerable to concussion injury. The flip side of the coin is that head trauma may serve as a triggering factor for migraines even in individuals who have never had a migraine. Care must be taken not to label a new migraine condition as persistent post-concussion syndrome.

TMJ: This is just a variation of the extra-cranial soft tissue injury mentioned above. TMJ stands for Temporo-mandibular Joint, which is the joint between the jaw and the skull. Trauma to the jaw can result in stretching injury and inflammation to the ligaments that hold these joints together. Malocclusion (misalignment of the teeth) by dislocation of the jaw can lead to further inflammation and pain in these regions often mistaken as "headache."

Benign Positional Vertigo: The inner ear is the balance organ that tells the brain how you are situated in space, sensing acceleration, and movement. Through a complex structure of tubes filled with liquid and crystals known as *otoliths*, the inner ear functions much like a carpenter's level. Traumatic forces to the head can lead to displacement of the otoliths in one or both ears. This results in misinformation of balance to the brain and results in vertigo. The vertigo is typically brief, lasting seconds, and less than a minute, but recurrent, brought on by further movement of the head. Recognition of this condition is very important because it is usually very easily treated with head rolling exercises such as *Epley* or *Semont* maneuvers.

Analgesic Overuse Headache: Also known as a "rebound headache," this is a well-known phenomenon amongst headache specialists whereby a medication is used to treat a headache disorder (traumatic or otherwise) and the chronic use of this medication leads to a new headache pattern that would not have happened if the medication was not used. These are usually milder, more diffuse headaches with a chronic daily pattern, typically not associated with nausea, light or sound sensitivity, or provoked by exertion.

Reactive Psychological Issues: Once concussed, life changes dramatically for the athlete. This person who has dedicated his life to physical activity is now told to go to physical and mental rest. School and work are missed. He may start falling behind in his obligations. The athlete's social structure may dramatically change. He may feel that he is letting his team, coaches, and family down by not being able to participate in his sport. These stressors may contribute to depressed mood, worry, and anger apart from the physiological changes in the brain.

Reactive Sleep Issues: Because the injured athlete is at rest, with low levels of arousal and may be sleeping during the day, or because of the emotional reactions described above, difficulty sleeping at night may occur. Nighttime sleep deprivation may in turn lead to daytime sleepiness and a vicious cycle of disturbed sleep ensues.

Cervical Strain/Sprain: Any time there is head injury, trauma to the neck, and spine must be considered. These injuries include strain and sprain of the muscles of the neck and ligaments associated with the spine. Fractures and dislocation of the vertebrae of the spine may also occur. These conditions can lead to headaches, and even vertigo, without direct injury to the brain.

Orthostatic Hypotension/Tachycardia: A rare condition that may occur after head injury is post-traumatic orthostatic hypotension/tachycardia. This condition occurs when blood pressure drops (hypotension) or the heart rate increases (tachycardia) abnormally when going from a lying to a standing position. Profound changes in these vital signs can lead to light-headedness and even fainting. Low-grade postural changes in these vitals can lead to a sense of chronic fatigue.

As you can begin to see, I believe concussions are beginning to emerge as a new field of science. As its mysteries unfold through research, I hope to capture key elements to understanding them, respecting their dangers, and providing recommendations for managing them within the context of sports. Concussions are receiving their moment in the spotlight, and for good reason. Now, let's take a closer look at the ways concussions occur and the resulting drain they cause on the brain.

## CHAPTER 5

BRAIN DRAIN

How Force Causes Concussions

Force equals mass times acceleration . . .
An object at rest tends to stay at rest until
acted on by an external force . . .
An object in motion tends to stay in motion
until acted on by an external force . . .
For every action there is an equal and opposite reaction . . .

The Physics of Concussion Injury

My personal experience dealing with symptoms from a concussion opened my eyes to the wonders contained within the brain. It's an organ of mystery and intrigue. Yet, the brain is ideally practical. Many areas of science study its fascinating powers to regulate all our bodily functions and behaviors. When working properly, the brain is a force to be reckoned with, able to drive individuals to succeed in all areas of life—physically, mentally, emotionally, socially, and spiritually.

When outside force is applied to the supple, and most important organ in the body, problems can occur. Memory can be forgotten. Emotions can be triggered. Impulsive decisions can be unleashed. Headaches can invade. Motivation can fade. Disabilities may develop. Some injuries have the capacity to alter a person's sense of self, while others affect abilities, such as speech or vision . . . and on the list goes.

The resulting "brain drain" is definitely another force to be reckoned with. It's important, therefore, to emphasize that I don't intend my term "brain drain" to be derogatory. I do not want to confuse brain drain with brain sprain, a phrase I use to relate to concussion and mild traumatic brain trauma. Instead, "drain," refers to reactions resulting in the brain when concussion occurs, due to increased struggle with supplying the metabolic demand for healing.

In this chapter, I'll provide guidance about the mechanisms and types of injury that cause concussions and more severe brain trauma. Additionally, I'll introduce an overview of some ways to see what's under the hood, speaking of various scanning modalities that shed light on how the brain is functioning and possible reasons for odd behaviors.

While the material will go into detail and introduce some medical terms, the goal is to give you a mini-neurology lesson so if you ever need to communicate with a doctor about a possible concussion, you will be better equipped to interpret the terminology related to the injury and ways to examine the brain. Trust me, this will merely scratch the surface of knowledge still being discovered today about the brain.

Breaking "It" Down

When I hurled head-first to tackle my friend, my head experienced the force of meeting oppositional inertia from my friend's hip. This caused a focal, and possibly angular impact injury to my prefrontal cortex, temporal lobes, and possibly my cerebellum. This resulted in an immediate electrolyte imbalance, a releasing of toxic excitatory neurotransmitters, such as "glutamate," and increased metabolic demand to assist with the cell recovery.

While these processes were occurring, I appeared dazed. Within a few minutes, my speech was impaired and my memory experienced retrograde and anterograde amnesia.

My brain had experienced a concussion, reeling to regain metabolic balance, a brain sprain that soon resulted in brain drain. ·

At this time, my brain immediately began assimilating and assisting in recovery upon receiving the force, my symptoms took time to develop, reaching a peak of impairment within an hour or two. After being taken to the Emergency Room, a computed tomography (CT) scan was ordered and results returned "normal" but clearly I was not acting normal.

Looking back, I realize now the doctor didn't have much concussion education. Although the CT scan was probably appropriate because of the sustained duration of my symptoms, admission to the hospital for observation was probably not warranted when the CT results returned normal. Within a few days, my symptoms subsided and fortunately, it appears my brain has healed.

To grasp the terminology used above, let's break down the mechanisms of injury before getting into more specific detail about what happens during a brain injury on a molecular level.

Mechanisms of Concussion Injury

Mechanisms refers to the ways the brain may be injured. You might think of a brain injury, or concussion, like a bruise to a banana. The exterior peel can only sustain so much pressure before the inside meat of the banana is bruised. The same goes for the brain and skull. Although the skull can sustain more forceful blows, the brain inside can become bruised, limiting the oxygen and blood flow in that particular area resulting in various symptoms. Unlike the banana, however, the brain can heal itself with proper health and lifestyle changes, or with certain medication intervention.

The skull does not have to suffer a blow for the brain to be injured.

> *It may be damaged immediately by the disruptive mechanical force of the impact or it may be affected some time later because of damage done to the skull. It is important to bear in mind that severe and even fatal damage to the brain may be sustained without significant injury to the scalp or skull.*

> *Conversely, extensive damage to the skull may be sustained without injury to the brain."*

Alan Moritz, M.D., Department of Legal Medicine, Harvard Medical School, "Mechanisms of Head Injury"

The most common mechanisms of brain injury in sports are:

- Player-player contact (70.3%)
- Player–playing surface contact (17.2%).

A concussion may occur in any or all of the following scenarios:

- Head-to-head contact
- Head-to-object contact
- Head-to-ground contact
- Head-to-body part contact
- Non-head contact due to sudden change in direction, e.g., whiplash.

Types of Contact

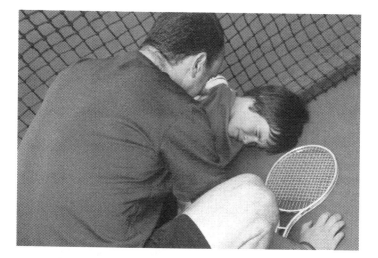

There are different types of contact that affect the brain. The following terms explain the differences, which also give insight to what symptoms may result. Additionally, understanding these types reveal that helmets may protect the skull, but do not protect the brain. There's no such thing as a "concussion-proof" helmets.

Focal Impact: Brain injury is located where the head was hit—point of contact.

Linear (or Translational): Brain injury that occurs as the brain moves within the skull. The brain sits inside the skull buoyed by fluid, and can slide back and forth. If there is enough force, like with a whiplash or focal impact, the brain can be injured on both the "coup" side and the "contra-coup" side.

Coup: The location where impact is received.

Contra-coup: The opposite side where the brain is damaged resulting from a recoil or counter movement. The contra-coup injury occurs when the brain "bounces back" from the focal location, injuring the opposite side. An example would be a hard fall that lands the player on their back. The back of the head slams the ground (coup, focal), and the brain's momentum immediately bounces forward to collide with the front area of the skull, affecting the prefrontal cortex.

Angular (or Rotational): Concussion resulting from a sudden head twist, causes shearing injury to the deeper tissues of the brain and to the brain stem.[2]

In my experience, rarely do concussions occur from only one mechanism of injury. Typically, they are realized in combination. The most common type of contact that results in concussion is when all three of these mechanisms are involved—focal, linear, and rotational.

---

[2]   Important Note: The rotational injury is the worst type of concussion injury, associated with the most serious neurological injuries.

Cognitive Neuroscience Emerges

As we dive deeper into the mechanisms of injury, you may appreciate knowing a bit about the origin of my particular area of specialty as it relates to understanding concussions and brain trauma.

I am among few neurologists in the world that study the physiology of the brain as it relates to behavior, forming a relatively new field of science called cognitive neurology. Cognitive neurology is ideally suited to study concussions because it is a clinical branch of neuroscience that overlaps disciplines related to the function and behavior of the brain resulting from injury or degeneration. Cognitive neuroscience looks at subsequent changes in the cognitive, emotional, and behavioral processes due to changes in neural circuitry.

Perhaps the first serious attempts to localize mental functions to specific locations of the brain was by French neurologist, Paul Broca, who studied how injury to the different parts of the brain effected psychological functions. In 1861, Broca worked with a man who was able to understand language but unable to speak. The man could only produce the sound "tan." It was later discovered that the man had damage to an area of his left frontal lobe now known as "Broca's area." This is one of the first cases to suggest a connection between physiological and specific behavioral changes.

The term *cognitive neuroscience* was not recognized as a unified discipline until the 1970s. Cognitive neuroscience began to integrate the newly laid theoretical ground in cognitive science that emerged between the 1950s and 1960s, with approaches in experimental psychology, neuropsychology, and neuroscience.

Pathophysiology

Pathophysiology explains the abnormal affects of a concussion or brain injury to the physiology of the brain. This is my particular area of specialty as a cognitive neurologist. Getting to the root-cause of concussions helps to understand the treatment options and ways to enhance the overall health of the brain. Let's look at traumatic injuries from macroscopic, microscopic, and molecular views:

Macroscopic

This refers to the tissue changes that occur with brain injury such as a concussion from a "naked eye" perspective:

Direct Trauma: Tissue changes resulting from direct trauma leads to traumatic brain injury. This is analogous to the fracture of a bone, the crush of a muscle, or the laceration of skin.

Cerebral Blood Flow: Changes to the volume of blood flow to brain tissue resulting from the trauma. This may lead to secondary ischemic injury or stroke, which are problems resulting from insufficient blood supply in more severe injury.

Hemorrhage (or Bleeding): Hemorrhage can occur in various regions. There is a leathery cover of the brain and spinal cord called the *dura*. Trauma can cause bleeding outside the dura called an *epidural hematoma*. These are usually caused by torn arteries, and so under high pressure, this kind of hemorrhage can lead to rapid and severe neurological deterioration and even death. Bleeding can occur under the dura, known as a *sub-dural hematoma*. These are usually due to tears of the veins, under much less pressure, with a slower deterioration, but could still lead to severe neurological impairment or even death. When bleeding occurs in the space immediately outside the surface of the brain, it is called a *subarachnoid hemorrhage*. When caused by trauma, subarachnoid hemorrhage is not usually fatal, but can be associated with neurological impairment, severe headache, and rarely a delayed spasm of the blood vessels that may lead to stroke. And finally, bleeding can occur within the tissue of the brain itself. This usually is like a bruise in the brain tissue associated with the direct tissue injury, or can be under pressure due to a torn blood vessel, where the pressure itself can cause further injury and become life threatening.

Microscopic

The microscopic view is much more important because many of the changes due to brain injury happen on a cellular level.

When the brain sustains an injury, the membranes of the brain cells stretch and lose their ability to regulate the environment of the cell. The membranes get "leaky" preventing the brain cells from working properly, leading to dysfunction which can affect behavior, concentration, memory, and other cognitive function.

Additionally, brain trauma increases the metabolic demand or energy necessary to repair the brain and regain the equilibrium inside the cell or neuron.

Molecular

Molecular brain trauma causes changes in the neurons, preventing the brain from working normally—including:

Inability to regulate electrolytes, which prevents the brain cells from operating properly. In the brain's natural or healthy state, the brain cell maintains the balance of salts and electrolytes inside and outside the cell. It takes energy to maintain that balance. When the brain is damaged, the membrane of the cell leaks out potassium while sodium leaks in. Therefore, the cell has to expend more energy to maintain this balance than before. The effect is the brain cell doesn't work properly in that particular region. For example, if brain damage and leaky electrolyte balance occurs in the area responsible for memory, then the result is short- and possibly long-term memory loss.

Releasing of toxic excitatory neurotransmitters such as *glutamate*, which is toxic to the cell. Although glutamate naturally occurs with proper brain function, when there's too much released as a result of brain trauma, then the results are dysfunction and further injury to the brain cells.

The concussion energy crisis: These injured neurons have a harder time getting enough sugar into the cells as they struggle to repair themselves and regain their equilibrium. The markedly increased demand for energy coupled with the reduction of available fuels leads to an energy crisis in the affected brain cells associated with brain dysfunction. Furthermore, with reduced blood flow, energy metabolism shifts from aerobic (using oxygen) to anaerobic metabolism resulting in a release of lactic acid. Lactic acid also can build up as a result of the trauma, which is further toxic to the brain cells (*local lactic acidosis*).[3]

Brain Mapping

If you break a bone, an X-ray can be ordered to see the break's location and severity. If you have chest pain, the doctor has a number of imaging options such as an MRI (magnetic resonance imaging), electrocardiogram (EKG), or echocardiogram, sonagram/ultrasound to help identify which organ is at fault. But it's not as simple to get a look at the brain. The brain, protected under 1–1.5cm of skull, is a multi-functional organ, so deciphering the injured location and resulting symptoms may require several imaging techniques.

Here's an overview of various types of "brain scans" and what you can expect should red flags of brain injury present after head trauma. I've also included a description of what I believe is the best technique to measure the brain's functions according to its anatomy. It's called *qEEG*, or *quantitative electroencephalography*.

CT: *Computed Tomography*, often referred to as a "cat" scan, is typically what the emergency room doctor will order if you bring in someone suspected of having a head injury. CT is a static imaging scan, featuring a computer-assisted method of assembling a "cross-section" X-Ray image of the brain. While the CT scan will reveal hemorrhaging, skull fractures,

---

[3]   Important Note: This is the main reason the brain needs rest immediately following a concussion is suspected. You don't want to add more metabolic demand to the brain during recovery.

and other structural abnormalities, it will not be able to distinguish the subtle changes resulting from a concussion.

MRI: *Magnetic Resonance Imaging* reveals the anatomy of the brain in greater detail than a CT and depicts a black-and-white virtual "section" of the brain. Using specialized techniques, an MRI may detect the shearing force injury and micro hemorrhages associated with concussion injury.

fMRI: *Functional Magnetic Resonance Imaging* is similar to that of MRI imaging. However, fMRI imaging takes advantage of a special property of tissue chemistry associated with metabolic activity. fMRI images provide scientists with both functional and anatomical information about brain tissue.

PET: *Positron Emission Tomography* allows scientists to view metabolic brain activity. PET works by measuring the distribution and movement of radioactively labeled molecules in the tissues of living subjects. The technique can be used to investigate changes in brain activity while the subject performs assigned tasks. Computers reconstruct PET scan data to produce two-dimensional or three-dimensional images. While MRI scans are used for research and in clinical settings for patient diagnosis, PET scans are used exclusively for research.

SPECT: Similar to PET, *Single-Photon Emission Computed Tomography* provides functional brain imaging, showing a three-dimensional view of the brain and measuring the blood flow and activity in the brain. It is cheaper than PET scans and does not require a cyclotron nearby to produce the necessary radioactive dyes.

qEEG: In my practice at Chesapeake Neurology Associates, and as Medical Director at Calvert Memorial Hospital in Maryland, I prefer using quantitative *Electroencephalography (qEEG)* to study brain physiology. This inexpensive technology measures electrical patterns at the surface of the scalp, which reflect cortical electrical activity in the brain. This real-time measurement records various "brainwaves" that we can measure accurately and map with statistical comparisons to normative populations, and therefore, localize areas of the brain that may be traumatized.

Cognitive Event Related Potentials

In the same way that PET, SPECT, and fMRI scans can be done while the subject is performing cognitive, thinking, and memory tasks, the electrical responses of the brain can also be measured and mapped to identify regions of dysfunction related to a specific cognitive task. Although this mapping lacks the spatial resolution that imaging studies such as MRI have, EEG analysis makes up for this with very high temporal resolution with ability to record events measured in milliseconds, rather than the several minutes required to do other imaging scans.

However, it's important to note that none of these imaging techniques serve as the ultimate or final answer to detecting a concussion. They may, however, serve critical roles in the assessment process to gather information for a specialist to make a diagnosis and a prognosis of recovery.

On the horizon, the sports world is beginning to see the concept of "bio markers" to help with detecting concussions. Using blood and saliva tests, we are continuing to learn that changes occurring in the brain may be apparent in these fluids.

According to a study published online in July 2014, in *JAMA Neurology*[4], blood levels of *total-tau*—a protein signaling axonal damage in the brain—could be used as a biomarker to gauge severity of concussions in athletes and to assess when it is safe to return to play. The study was conducted by a team led by Pashtun Shahim, MD, PhD, of Sahlgrenska University Hospital, Molndal, Sweden.

"T-tau is a promising biomarker for the diagnosis and prognosis of concussion in athletes," Dr. Shahim commented to Medscape Medical News.[5] "I would say if you suspect concussion, you could measure blood levels of T-tau, and then repeat the test every few days to gauge whether it is safe to go back to play."

---

[4]   Pashtun Shahim, MD; Kaj Blennow, MD, PhD; and Henrik Zetterberg, MD, PhD, *Tau, S-100 Calcium-Binding Protein B, and Neuron-Specific Enolase as Biomarkers of Concussion—Reply*, JAMA Neurology, (American Medical Association, July 2014), as appears on the Internet at http://archneur.jamanetwork.com/article.aspx?articleid=1886221&resultClick=3.

[5]   Sue Hughes, *Blood Biomarker for Concussion Identified* (Medscape Medical News: Neurology, March 26, 2014). Interview of Dr. Shahim published online March 13, 2014, by JAMA Neurol, http://www.medscape.com/viewarticle/822579.

He added: "Our data is very promising but it needs to be replicated in a larger sample size before we can recommend this approach for routine use. In future, there could be a point-of-care test that could be used at the side of the pitch."

The study showed that the plasma levels of T-tau increased in ice hockey players with sports-related concussion. The highest concentrations of T-tau were measured immediately after the injury, and the levels declined during the first 12 hours, followed by a second peak between 12 and 36 hours. Importantly, T-tau concentrations at one hour after concussion predicted the number of days it took for the concussion symptoms to resolve and the players to return to play safely.

Additionally, researchers at George Mason are comparing preseason samples of saliva to the samples from kids who suffered head injuries. They think the change in saliva proteins after a concussion may become a non-invasive way to identify the presence of a concussion.

As you can see, diagnosing a concussion and traumatic brain injuries is not a cut-and-dry process.

The sports world may be more familiar with the term "baseline" tests, involving neuro-cognitive performance measures prior to the season. Performing baseline tests on all athletes should be a requirement, in my opinion. During the season, in the event of a suspected concussion, the athlete can retake the neuro-cognitive test, and the scores can be compared, revealing tangible data that can help in assessing the risk of concussion. I created my own baseline test, which is integrated into a comprehensive platform for concussion management. Details about this protocol are in Chapter 8.

## CHAPTER 6

BRAIN DRAMA

Concussion Repercussions

When the brain meets enough force to cause it to bump against the inside of the skull, a variety of short-term symptoms can arise. And unfortunately, long-term and dangerous consequences can develop as well. A concussion, considered to be a mild traumatic brain injury (mTBI), can either: heal quickly (seven days to 12 months); or, be the starting point of future problems; as well as, complicate existing brain-health issues that accelerate the onset of more serious conditions, neurological disorders, and other brain drama.

The brain is a particularly sensitive organ making awareness of concussion repercussions serious business. I believe a common misconception is that after an athlete appears to have recovered from a concussion or substantial hit to the head, they are "back to normal." While the initial symptoms may have subsided, the brain may be affected forever, akin to a "scar" that blemishes the skin after healing from a scrape, cut, or other surface wound. Perhaps more accurately, a concussion could be compared to internal ligament damage of a sprain that when "healed," residual scarring can impede movement, restrict flexibility, and reduce overall performance capabilities.

While the concussion symptoms may have subsided, look out for other odd behaviors, impulsive decisions, personality changes, anger outbursts, emotional imbalances, memory difficulties—all of which signal problematic neurological disorders resulting from brain damage.

In my practice, I treat patients dealing with a wide variety of symptoms, sleep problems, and behaviors. As I begin the initial assessment process, one of the first questions I ask is, "Have you ever been hit in the head?"

While most psychiatrists and therapists typically examine behaviors from a psychological point of view—like understanding triggers anchored from past abuse, traumatic events, heredity, etc.—as a cognitive neurologist I dig for physiological changes to the brain that may be the root cause of the behavior.

By understanding the overall "health" of the brain, then I can recommend interventions with medication, natural remedies, and lifestyle changes. Working in tandem with a psychiatrist or therapist, we can improve the physical health of the brain, as well as give the patient new strategies to deal, improve, or change related undesirable behaviors that I call "brain drama."

In this chapter, I want to increase your sensitivity to the serious consequences of concussions and resulting possibilities of brain damage. First, let's start with addressing the most serious decision in sports—when should you allow a suspected concussed athlete to return to play?

Two-Minute Warning

From the moment an athlete sustains a hit that bumps the brain against the inner table of the skull the clock starts ticking. The next few minutes that follow lead to the most serious decision in sports. During this period, a number of neurological, physiological, financial, and perhaps philosophical, repercussions occur, perhaps with life or death hanging in the balance.

Onlookers may be gasping or cheering with the sound of collision. Amidst opponent's trash-talking, teammates and coaches may be eagerly helping the player to their feet. The athlete who sustained the hit immediately begins self-assessing their ability to return to play, tasking the potentially-injured brain and body to cooperate and signals its own concussion pass or fail test.

Unfortunately, the athlete is not the best judge to make this decision. Nor are the coaches. Conflicts of interest abound. Hopefully, an athletic trainer or team doctor intervenes and carries out a series of assessments to help identify the severity of a concussion risk. Then typically, the decision is made—play or sit.

It's this period of time, from the hit to the return-to-play decision, where I fear sports may be risking too much. Too often, the post-hit evaluation process is rushed. While all eyes are on the scoreboard, not enough emphasis is on the future well-being of the athlete.

Complicating matters further, signs of a concussion often take several minutes, hours, or even days to materialize.

Science continues to discover ways of assessing concussions. Numerous studies show a connection between brain trauma and problematic futures. Consider these:

- Almost half of homeless men had traumatic brain injuries (http://www.sciencedaily.com/releases/2014/04/140425104714.htm).
- Teenagers who have had a concussion also have higher rates of suicide attempts (http://www.sciencedaily.com/releases/2014/04/140415181325.htm).
- Head injuries can make children loners (http://www.sciencedaily.com/releases/2014/04/140410083505.htm).
- Teen concussions increase risk of depression (http://www.sciencedaily.com/releases/2014/01/140109175502.htm).

Perhaps an even louder wake-up call is that most concussions are not reported, and overt concussions are not required to cause brain damage. A 2012 study by the American Association of Neurological Surgeons, looked at 45 high school varsity football players, none of who experienced a clinical concussion during the season. The researchers concluded a single season of football play can produce measurable brain changes that have been previously associated with mTBI—"adding to the increasing amounts of literature demonstrating that a season of participation in a contact sport can show changes in the brain in the absence of concussion or clinical findings."[6]

Another grave concern is the condition known as *Second Impact Syndrome*, or sudden cerebral swelling that may occur when a second concussion occurs while the brain is recovering from injury. Most people don't realize the 50 percent fatality rate among individuals who suffer this fortunately rare event. Of the survivors, 100 percent will have permanent neurological impairments.

Then there is the more common *Post-Concussion Syndrome (PCS)*. This condition results in various symptoms that may persist for days, weeks, months, or even years causing complications with the quality of life. PCS symptoms may include:

- Physical fatigue
- Dizziness/vertigo, nausea
- Headaches (sensitivity to light, sound)
- Sleep disturbances (difficulty sleeping, staying awake or excessive daytime sleeping)
- Emotional impairment (personality changes, irritability, anxiety, depression)
- Cognitive impairment (aka: "brain fog" typically involving recent or short-term memory loss, poor attention and concentration)

Another seemingly obvious realization is that the hit that may have caused concussion-like symptoms, was not the first. In fact, if the athlete participated in practice, particularly in American football, the head had sustained numerous, if not thousands of *sub-concussive* hits prior to the one that caused the symptomatic blow.

Then, think of all the other times the individual was hit in the head previously in life during other activities like skiing, cycling, falls at a young age, fist-fighting, or in other sports and you can begin to see a straw that's about to break the camel's back. When the brain suffers a hit,

[6] American Association of Neurological Surgeons (AANS), *Brain Changes Can Result from Participation In One Year of Contact Sports, Evidence Shows.* (April 8, 2014). http://www.sciencedaily.com/releases/2014/04/140408154105.htm.

but symptoms do not arise, we call them *asymptomatic* or sub-concussive, because slight damage may have been caused but not felt.

These series of repetitive hits cumulatively may lead to *Chronic Traumatic Encephalopathy* (CTE), which is a progressive degenerative disease of the brain found in athletes with a history of repetitive brain trauma, including symptomatic concussions as well as asymptomatic sub-concussive hits to the head.

Autopsies reveal CTE is associated with a build-up of Tau protein, and looks like a brain afflicted by Alzheimer's disease. CTE, the focus of the current NFL lawsuits among active and former players, may also be affected by lifestyle factors that can add stress to the damaged brain, including smoking, alcohol abuse, drug use, poor diet, and lack of exercise. Medical science has not yet fully uncovered why some athletes develop CTE, while others don't.

Another frightful symptom that may result from a concussion is the appearance of *seizures*. Seizures typically occur immediately upon losing consciousness or within the first week of the injury. Seizures are physical manifestations resulting from abnormal electrical discharges in the brain. These manifestations appear to be convulsions—when the body shakes rapidly, even violently.

Seizures occur in about 5 percent of head injuries, and usually within the first seven days. They typically occur more often when hits create a skull fracture or cerebral contusion, and occur more often in adults. Here are the most typical seizure risk factors after mTBI:

- Post traumatic amnesia lasting longing than 12 hours
- Intracranial bleeding
- Persistent neurologic deficit
- Skull fracture

Perhaps one of the more devastating potential repercussions of brain injury is the damage to the central nervous system, leading to *paralysis*. Our nervous system is especially sensitive to damage by injury. Both brain and spinal cord injuries have the potential to cause severe and life-changing disabilities. However, the type of disability sustained depends greatly on the region of trauma. The spinal cord is responsible for information transfer between the brain and the body. It follows that injuries to the spinal cord disrupt information transfer. The position of trauma to the spine largely determines the effect of a spinal cord injury on the body. For instance, injuries to the lower half of the spine can lead to *paraplegia* (paralysis of the lower half of the body with involvement of both legs), while injuries in the neck or brainstem may lead to *quadriplegia* (paralysis of both arms and both legs). Injury to one side of the brain may lead to *hemiplegia* of the opposite side of the body.

Is this nervous system damage completely avoidable? In theory, yes. Realistically, no. Risk can be mitigated, especially during the moments following a suspected concussion.

Tips for Dealing with Decision to Return to Play

It's a scary moment to see an athlete laying on the ground for any reason. Most bone breaks, muscle tears, and sprains will heal in time. Every brain is different. Every athlete has had different lifestyles. Every hit to the head can have life-long consequences. In Chapter 8, we will get into detail about a comprehensive approach to managing concussions from pre-season through the career of the athlete. Before rushing to get the athlete back in the game, the following precautionary steps are appropriate:

1. Don't move the unconscious person.

In the event of loss of consciousness, don't attempt to move the unresponsive individual and risk exacerbating the problem of a neck and spinal cord injury. During a loss of consciousness, the brain and body are experiencing a forced re-boot, but the person's pulse and breathing should continue. The unconscious athlete should be assumed to have a spinal injury until proven otherwise. Should the individual stay unconscious for longer than a minute, call for help.

2. Better to wait, than be sorry.

A loss of consciousness may be the most obvious symptom, but also not likely to occur. Only one in 10 concussions result in a loss of consciousness. Therefore, onlookers have to be highly tuned into possible signs of a concussion. Symptoms can vary depending on the individual and where the brain suffers trauma. Generally, one should be aware of a glazed-over look in the eyes, headache, vomiting, vertigo, and perhaps signs of confusion within a few seconds.

If there is any hint of these, I recommend asking the athlete if they can stand and walk/skate to the sideline unassisted. Now, the waiting game begins. The athlete should rest a few minutes before conducting any concussion assessments. Record and report the results and wait again. Don't let the athlete, or coach, try to talk them back into action.

I've created a protocol to help with the on-the-field concussion assessment. It involves cognitive, emotional, and balance measures using a mobile app on a smartphone. It guides the responsible person on the sideline through a step-by-step process of assessing memory, orientation, and balance for a potentially injured athlete and instantly documents and reports the results. This tool is a companion to a comprehensive concussion management platform. More on this in Chapter 8.

3. Wait some more.

The least popular decision is to wait and observe. During this period of time, the brain is rapidly trying to restore itself, flooding blood and oxygen to the injury. Other functions may be compromised. Decision-making could be influenced. Further injury to the brain is the enemy, not the opponent on the field. Sometimes, concussion symptoms show up the next day. So, even if the athlete passes the sideline assessment, unless a trained medical professional has determined that there was no concussion, just the suspicion that a concussion may have occurred warrants that the player sit out for the rest of the day.

4. Allow for recovery.

A recovery protocol needs to be set into motion. It begins with rest, minimizing mental, and physical stimulation until the athlete is symptom free. The concept is *relative rest*, meaning the avoidance of any mental or physical activity that provokes the athlete's concussion-related symptoms. Once the injured player is free of symptoms at rest, I have included a "5-step Progressive Exertion Recovery Guide" built into my protocol that monitors symptoms, and guides the timeline for a return to practice or even classroom activities.

5. Decide.

Notice how carefully I'm recommending a hard hit should be treated? A decision to allow a player to return to the game too soon, has too many risks. Give it time. Give it rest. Follow a recovery protocol, monitor symptoms, and then decide when to return.

The Public Broadcasting Service television program, "Frontline," has been tracking concussions during the last two seasons of the National Football League (NFL). Among the alarming discoveries, 49.5 percent of players never missed a game after sustaining a concussion. Given that the average concussion injury takes 10 to 14 days of recovery, I feel many of these players may be returning to the game too soon.

While there is no standard recovery time from a concussion, guidelines from the American Academy of Neurology and endorsed by the NFL Players Association, find that athletes are at the greatest risk of repeat injury in the first 10 days post-concussion. And research suggests that the more head injuries a person suffers, the more likely they are to suffer from *Chronic Traumatic Encephalopathy* (CTE) and face complications later in life.

The bottom line is that awareness and patience helps the athlete avoid becoming an unfortunate statistic.

Repercussion Facts

These additional facts and factors affect the return-to-play decision. Consider:

- The younger the athlete, the more vulnerable the brain is to concussion, and will require longer recovery periods. The brain continues developing through the age of 25. Therefore, concussions in our youth and collegiate athletes, can result in greater damage and risk of cognitive impairment.
- A concussed athlete is more likely to sustain a repeat concussion, with the greatest risk in the first seven days.
- Repeat concussions are slower to recover.
- Athletes who have sustained three or more concussions are likely to have long-term cognitive impairment and emotional struggles.
- Concussions can accelerate the onset of dementia and Alzheimer's disease.
- People with a history of migraines are more vulnerable to concussion injury.

Repercussion Factors

Unfortunately, when the brain is injured, the injury causes malfunction. While concussions are a milder form of brain injury, a number of factors influence how well the brain heals and what functions may be altered. As the brain grapples to return to normalcy, it often builds alternate paths for the neural signaling to occur. This can result in a change in performance, which can appear to be a change in someone's personality.

Some factors that influence the lasting impression concussions may have include:

Heredity: Genetic history of neurological disorders can be passed down. Although these genetic profiles do not automatically guarantee a future of disorder, they can have an influence. Heredity can also influence the vulnerability or susceptibility to develop neurological conditions.

Gender: A number of studies have identified that women are more vulnerable to concussion injury than men. In any sport (such as soccer) where women compete with the same rules as men, the incidence of concussion injury is greater. A variety of factors have been postulated as contributors to this phenomenon. Women have smaller neck sizes, making the head more likely to "whiplash." About 20 percent of women suffer from migraines. And women are more likely to express concerns about their health than men.

Pre-Natal Health: The health of your brain directly relates to health of your mother during pregnancy, particularly during the first trimester. During this phase, the human brain development is largely based on the level of nutrition, exercise, and psychological condition of the mother. Alcohol, smoking tobacco, and drug use during pregnancy can inhibit brain development, which can have negative affects on the whole neurological system in the future.

History of Migraines: Individuals with a history of migraines are more vulnerable to post-concussion symptoms than those without.

Previous Brain Injury: One concussion offers enough risk for the future. When they add up, then the brain begins to work around the problem areas. This may lead to heightened risk of erratic behavior or cognitive impairment. Any previous brain injury, whether it was diagnosed, perceptible, or recognized, can lead to future problems.

Lifestyle: The future health of your brain is made of the past (heredity, pre-natal health and previous brain injury), but also the present. The lifestyle, or in other words, how well someone takes care of his or her health, can affect future risk of impairment. Some of those factors include:

- **Nutritious Foods** — Diets void of healthy carbohydrates, protein, and water can leave the brain gasping for nutrition critical for proper cellular development and operation.
- **Exercise** — We often assume athletes lead a life with regular exercise. However, it's not always the case, particularly after the

playing years. Low levels of exercise reduce blood flow to the brain creating vulnerability to injury.

- **Sleep** — Rejuvenating restful, deep sleep is required for the brain to work optimally. Low levels of sleep force the brain to work harder than necessary to perform normal functions. When brain injury occurs, the brain may be at a deficit already due to lack of sleep, which can extend the healing period and risk of impairment.

- **Alcohol** — Drinking alcohol alters the brain chemistry, affects memory and leaves a toxic or poisonous presence that reduces overall brain function. Alcohol is a neurotoxin. But perhaps most concerning is, the brain cannot heal as well from injury when there are residual affects of too much alcohol.

- **Drug Use** — Illegal drug use is not only highly addictive, and leads to bad decisions, but drugs also leave toxic elements in the brain that "weaken" the brain's ability to operate properly. The more drugs are present, the easier a brain can be damaged from blunt trauma such as a concussion.

- **Smoking Tobacco** — Not only does nicotine affect memory negatively, but tobacco is loaded with many additives and carcinogens, which are also toxic to the brain. Like alcohol and drug use, a toxic brain is more susceptible to the effects of concussion injury.

- **Environment** — The polluted air we breathe, the contaminated water we drink, and toxins found in foods can impact our brain health. For example, fumes from paint, nail polish, and hair dye and perms, if absorbed frequently, can reduce your brain's ability to heal quickly.

Cognitive and Emotional Impairments

Other than paralysis or dying from complications suffered from brain trauma, the most serious concussion repercussion is a significant decrease in overall quality of life. This may be due to headaches and a variety of cognitive and emotional impairments that develop as a post-concussion syndrome. Memory loss, poor attention span, and improper decision-making are warning signs of brain-related trouble. An estimated 50-million Americans suffer from disorders of the brain or nervous system, which is a pretty good sized chunk of the 317-million population. Some brain disorders are influenced by genetics, some are environmental, others from spinal cord or brain injury; and some result from a combination of any or all of these factors.

Traumatic brain injury (TBI) refers to damage resulting from trauma to the brain. TBI, like spinal cord injuries, may result in impaired physical function. However, the brain not only controls our sensory and motor functions, it is also our center of conscious thought. Therefore, injuries to the brain can affect our cognitive abilities or disturb behavioral and emotional functioning. In addition, brain trauma has the potential to alter personality, and the sense of "self."

TBI by Region

Trauma to different regions of the brain results in different types of disabilities. Some injuries have the capacity to alter a person's sense of self, while others affect abilities such as speech or vision but do not affect a person's sense of who they are. Functional imaging has greatly aided the ability to locate the region of the brain responsible for behavior.

When you play a contact sport, you may be trading cognitive function for the thrill of game—playing Russian roulette with your future. From a medical perspective, playing contact sports is not a healthy or wise risk. Although you may enjoy sport and realize there are many benefits of the game and being on a team, I caution you with the conditions that are to follow below that can result if the gamble goes wrong.

In my practice, I avoid using "labels" for various conditions, preferring to understand the physiological issue causing the symptoms. Nevertheless, I've grouped a number of cognitive and emotional impairments that may occur should a concussion, or repeated sub-concussive hits lead to degenerative brain or neurological damage (in alphabetical order):

Alzheimer's Disease: Researchers believe Alzheimer's and other forms of dementia actually start decades before people experience their first symptoms. This may, in part, have to do with related brain trauma.

Alzheimer's is a progressive, degenerative brain disease that leads to loss of cognitive function and short- and long-term memory, behavioral changes, personality changes, and impaired judgment. Typically affecting the temporal and parietal lobes, the brains of Alzheimer's patients also contain tangled masses of abnormal protein in the cerebrum.

A recent study conducted at the Mayo Clinic Study of Aging in Pittsburgh, reported in the scientific journal *Neurology*, there is evidence of a link between concussions and Alzheimer's disease. The conclusion stated:

> *Among individuals with mild cognitive impairment, but not cognitively normal individuals, self-reported head trauma with at least momentary loss of consciousness or memory was associated with greater amyloid deposition, suggesting that head trauma may be associated with Alzheimer disease–related neuropathology.* [7]

Anxiety: Anxiety is an emotional response from over-anticipation of a real or perceived future threat, according to the *Diagnostic and Statistical Manual of Mental Disorders, 5th Edition* (DSM-V). People can experience anxiety when the cingulate gyrus, area of the brain surrounding the deep limbic system, is damaged. The basal ganglia helps to integrate thoughts, feelings, and movements, as well as help set and interpret anxiety levels. This area is also involved with experiencing feelings of pleasure. Problems associated with the cingulate can be related to struggles with stress, anxiety, and related symptoms such as insomnia, stomachaches, and muscle tension.

Attention Deficit: New research suggests brain injury may also be a cause of attention deficit disorder. This can come about following exposure to toxins or physical injury. Experts say that head injuries can cause ADD-like symptoms in previously unaffected people, perhaps due to frontal lobe damage resulting in impairment of executive functioning. However, further research connecting brain trauma with attention deficit is needed.

---

[7]   Michelle M. Mielke, PhD and others, *Head Trauma and in Vivo Measures of Amyloid and Neurodegeneration in a Population-Based Study*, published online before print December 26, 2013, http://www.neurology.org/content/early/2013/12/26/01.wnl.0000438229.56094.54.short.

The DSM-V describes attention deficit as a persistent pattern of inattention that interferes with functioning and development, characterized by inability to give close attention to details, difficulty sustaining attention in tasks, inability to listen when spoken to directly, inability to follow through on instructions, failing to finish work, and difficulty organizing tasks and activities—especially sequential tasks. More succinctly put, it's the inability to focus your thoughts and attention.

Balance: Sometimes traumatic brain injury can cause **balance** and **equilibrium** problems. Balance problems after head trauma can fall under either *peripheral* or *central injuries*. Central injuries refer to injury of the central nervous system structures having to do with balance and coordination including the cerebellum and the brainstem. Peripheral injuries refer to injury to the inner ear structure or Cranial Nerve VIII, which is the cranial nerve that carries information from the ear (including the inner ear) to the brain. There are also issues, which are considered sensory problems, as they are associated with the parts of the brain that govern vision and hearing. Midline shift syndrome, in which balance and equilibrium are affected, generally goes hand-in-hand with *post-trauma vision syndrome*. Symptoms of midline shift syndrome and other balance disorders include:

- Continual sense of disequilibrium
- Difficulty maintaining balance
- Incorrect weight distribution and posture
- Inappropriate gait
- Trouble walking in a straight line

Patients of midline shift syndrome frequently also complain that the walls seem to be moving in on them or the horizon is oddly tilted.

Behavior Problems: Symptoms of brain injury can appear in a wide range of previously rare behavior. Examples include:

- Aggression toward others
- Aggression toward self
- Tantrums and crying

- Yelling and cursing
- Explosive anger
- Non-compliance
- Property destruction

Bipolar: A mood disorder somewhere on the spectrum between depression and schizophrenia is marked by severe fluctuation of manic episodes. Several studies have shown a link between people with bipolar and other psychiatric disorders with head trauma.

Brain Fog: Brain fog refers to a low degree of delirium where the brain is sluggish with its function. Sometimes called "clouding of consciousness," it can be manifested in a wide range of general daily activities, affecting short-term memory, and ability to focus and calculate decisions. It's similar to the feeling of being sleep deprived for a few days or experiencing a severe hangover.

Chronic Fatigue: When the brain is injured, it requires a lot of fuel and energy to heal and find ways to return to normal operation. The unfortunate byproduct can be a sense of fatigue during typical daily activities. Long-term studies are few with this condition, but logic would attribute poor brain health with lack of overall energy, and susceptibility to decline unless medical or lifestyle changes intervene. At least one study showed head trauma is a common trigger of chronic fatigue as well as fibromyalgia.

Cognitive Difficulty: Cognitive issues are any issue related to thinking. These problems can be relatively mild and can improve over time, or they can be more severe, long-term issues that make it difficult for the survivor to live independently. Cognitive thinking includes being aware of one's surroundings, being able to pay attention, concentrate, short-term memory, reasoning, problem solving, and executive skills such as goal setting, planning, initiating, self-awareness, and self-monitoring and evaluation. Typically cognitive difficulty arises from trauma to the frontal lobes, or prefrontal cortex.

Comorbidity: In psychiatry, psychology, and mental health counseling, comorbidity refers to the presence of more than one diagnosis occurring in an individual at the same time. However, in psychiatric classification, comorbidity does not necessarily imply the presence of multiple diseases, but instead can reflect our current inability to supply a single diagnosis that accounts for all symptoms.

Depression: Prolonged sadness may be a symptom of any number of circumstances in life, brain health included. A brain diminished in functioning either from concussion, severely shaken, other trauma, or degenerative disease may not have normal aptitude for resilience to deal with events of life.

Language and Speech: Language-related difficulties can develop from traumatic brain injury. Problems can be the result of damage to areas that govern communication in the brain, or they can be the result of motor problems or weaknesses. Examples include various forms of *Aphasia*, which affects both comprehension and production of speech, as well as the ability to read and write. Language difficulties relating to motor problems include:

- *Apraxia* — Exhibited with difficulty coordinating mouth and speech movements; and,
- *Dysarthria* — The individual can think of the right words to use, but neurological damage prevents him or her from using the muscles needed to form the words.

Memory and Learning: Immediate recall, otherwise known as "short-term" as well as "long-term" memory, which refers to information stored for extended durations, may be affected by brain trauma. Thought to be like a super-computer with files of information, the brain stores memories much differently, typically encoding neural connections giving the brain the ability to recall information and experiences. Memory and learning are related, and remains a fascinating subject of research. Still, we know memory fades over time, and memory loss may be accelerated by brain trauma, and lifestyle.

Parkinson's Disease: Another human brain disorder that may be connected to brain trauma is *Parkinsonuman brain*, a motor system disorder affecting more than 500,000 Americans. A study conducted in 2011 by the University of California, Los Angeles (UCLA) researchers, found that while a traumatic brain injury does not cause Parkinson's, it can make individuals more susceptible to the neurodegenerative disorder that affects roughly 1 to 2 percent of the population over the age of 65.

The disease is characterized by tremor, rigidity, slowness of movement, and impaired balance and coordination. It occurs when neurons in certain sections of the midbrain die or become impaired. The neuronal loss causes a decrease in the level of an excitatory neurotransmitter, which causes the neurons in another part of the brain to initiate aberrant neural impulses. Genetic factors may play a stronger role in some forms of the disease, while environmental factors play a primary role in other forms.

Sleep Disorders: Humans require sleep to rejuvenate and brain trauma may interfere with that process resulting in fatigue felt in the brain and body. My practice has taken sleep very seriously, treating patients with sleep apnea, fatigue, restless leg syndrome, chronic insomnia, and narcolepsy. Without deep sleep, the brain and body malfunctions, like an engine without fuel. Concussions can affect sleep negatively, which is ironically the best way to heal from the trauma.

Hopefully by now, you see repercussions of concussions can be deadly, dangerous and can start or exacerbate any number of pre-existing conditions with sad long-term impairments. The next time you hear someone say "you got your bell rung," it won't illicit casual banter about being tough and getting back in the game. Instead, you'll take it as serious as a heart attack.

Unfortunately, the sports world and sports culture is partly to blame for the slew of athletes who return to the game with a brain knocked silly. In the next chapter, we'll investigate modern sports culture, how politicians are stepping in to help, and concussion treatment challenges that are putting our athletes at risk.

## CHAPTER 7

THE SPORTS CULTURE PARADIGM SHIFT

Are We Developing Mental Toughness or Breeding Concussions?

Sports provide many opportunities for athletes to learn about teamwork, knowing roles, leadership, promptness, attention, dedication, loyalty, hard work, commitment, overcoming adversity, how to win, how to lose, sportsmanship, physical fitness, as well as learning about themselves. Sports are the ultimate entertainment for players because they can exercise their talents, gifts, and abilities within the framework of team competition and a season. Then they can see the fruits of their labor, even with a losing season.

Sports also provide players a vehicle to learn about mental and physical toughness, which is a powerful intangible attribute to carry into life off the playing surface. Being "tough" is an important and valuable asset. But when does toughness, and the culture that breeds it, cross the line?

When an athlete breaks a bone, sprains an ankle, tears a ligament or suffers virtually any other visible injury, they are helped off the field to begin the healing and rehabilitating process. There's no shame in getting injured. Instead these injuries foster empathy, concern and perhaps even increased awareness of the risks of playing the game.

But when an athlete suffers a hit to head or hard fall, they stumble to their feet and are typically encouraged to "walk it off" and "tough it out."

Despite momentary confusion, perhaps a dazed, vacant stare the athlete often "digs deep" to stay in the game (or practice) with the illusion that it's benefiting the team. If they pull themselves out of the game for this "invisible injury," they fear they will be called "soft" or "weak," ultimately feeling guilt and shame for not being tough enough, and letting the team down.

While sports can be an excellent teacher, the sports culture may be the biggest culprit of breeding concussions, sub-concussions, brain trauma and problems later in life resulting from cognitive and emotional impairment.

When it comes to concussions, we need to realize developing mental toughness doesn't mean you play with a brain injury.

In this chapter, let's look at the cultural elements of sports that may be increasing or decreasing the concussion risk—from inside the huddle, locker room, and training room to legislation, equipment and even the White House. By understanding the psychological and sociological dynamics, I hope to be a catalyst of cultural change that's required with everyone involved in the game.

Implicit or Explicit Acceptance of Risk

Everyone knows there is risk to contact and collision sports. Even sports and recreational activities that don't involve contact have a certain amount of risk. Every time a person gets on a bicycle, or a skateboard, or runs on to the field of play, that person is aware of the fact that injury may occur. For adult athletes, there is a clear understanding that engaging in sports and recreational activities may result in injury that can result in long-term disability and even death.

But who, in our society, is responsible for disseminating the information to those athletes about what the risks really are? It is generally assumed that the adult athlete is mature enough to seek out the knowledge and awareness of these risks before taking them on. It is also assumed that those in our society that are aware of these risks have a moral and ethical obligation to impart that knowledge to those that don't.

What about the youth athlete? The brains of children and teenagers have not developed fully. This may result in more impulsive risk taking behavior than an person with a fully mature brain may engage in. Modern society does not allow minors to make serious legal, financial or medical decisions on their own. Who then is responsible for the "informed consent" of our youth as they take the field? Of course, it is their parent or guardian's responsibility to know and understand the risks of injury, both short- and long-term before allowing their child to participate in any sport, and this applies especially to concussion injury.

The risk of playing sports comes with many conflicts of interest as well.

Conflicts of Interest

The athlete wants to play. The athlete's teammates want the athlete to play. The coach wants the athlete to play. The parents want the athlete to play. The athletes are surrounded by a village of "conflicts of interest."

The sports world glamorizes athletes who "play through injury," cheering when an athlete shows the grit and determination to serve the team's competitive goal. Herein is our first conflict of interest. The enthusiasm created by the fans, combined with the desire to play and win the game and perhaps notoriety, conflict with the reality that playing injured drastically increases the odds of sustaining further damage.

While being tough-minded is an important aspect of sports, we need to push a new agenda that replaces the culture to "win at all costs."iThe physical and mental health of an athlete is far more valuable than a checkmark in the win column.

This is particularly true with regard to concussions. Any player suspected of having a concussion, should be immediately removed from activity for evaluation and observation. While the athlete may be mentally tough, the brain is not, and traumatic brain injury has dangerous, serious short- and long-term side effects.

My biggest concern is the next conflict of interest virtually everybody has with wanting the athlete to play as soon as possible, instead of allowing enough time and healing to occur. Greater emphasis needs to be on protecting the athletes' well-being long-term, instead of rushing the athlete to gameplay hoping the athlete "will be fine."

In other words, every time an athlete suffers a potential concussion, the future of our country and economy is at stake. Penalties should be levied on teams who allow athletes to play injured, and return to action too soon.

Who then can be the advocate for the athlete's brain?

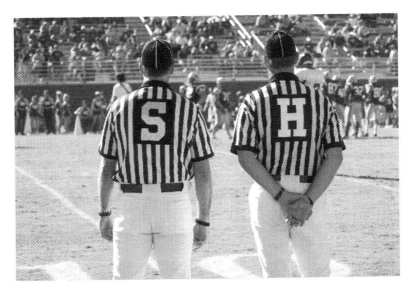

There are a couple of obvious choices. On the field the one unbiased person that is closest to the athletes as they collide is the referee or the umpire. This person should be the most objective observer when it comes to witnessing the collision and the behavior of the potentially injured player. Rules of the game should include the authority of the referee to single out a potentially injured athlete and send them out for a sideline assessment. The professional organizations of referees and umpires should take a leadership role in ensuring that their members are educated on the recognition of the signs of concussion injury and awareness of the potential short term and long term consequences of allowing an athlete to continue playing after concussion injury.

Ideally, the medical professional on the sidelines is ethically obligated to prioritize the health of the athlete's brain over the pressure applied by coaches, team owners, parents and any other individuals pushing to get the athlete back into the game. Unfortunately, this is often not the case. In the professional sports world, team doctors are paid by the team, and there in lies another potential conflict of interest. The current NFL Protocol for concussion injury has adjusted for this by including an independent concussion specialist on the sideline and during the recovery period, however, this policy falls short as the ultimate decision as to whether a concussion has occurred or not, and whether a player has recovered sufficiently to return to the game is retained by the team doctor. Furthermore, the NFL protocol includes an "eye in the sky" with athletic trainers able to review instant replay video to detect collisions that may have resulted on concussion.

Changing these conflicts of interest means changing priorities, such as:

- Athletes' dream of fame and fortune — OR — Athletes' dream of a long, healthy life.
- Coaches desire for winning records — OR — Coaches' desire for players retiring in good health.
- Parents' hopes for athletic scholarships — OR — Parents' hopes for academic scholarship.
- Team owners to make money — OR — Team owners who invest in players' futures.

Legal and ethical issues abound as these unique features of sport related concussion injury are taken into account. The common thread to the solution to the issues that are raised by acceptance of risk, risk compensation, cultural minimization, and conflicts of interest is the imperative need to place the health of the athlete's brain as the top priority over gameplay by everyone involved, including the athlete

It Takes a Village

Borrowing this phrase from Senator Hillary Clinton, changing sports culture will need to involve everyone affiliated with the game. When it comes to concussions, everyone needs to assume appropriate responsibility, despite conflicts of interest. For example:

Athletes: It begins with the player who must have heightened awareness of the concussion risks, who respects sportsmanlike conduct and follows concussion management protocol to return to practice and gameplay safely. Goals of a professional athletic career or earning an athletic scholarship must have the condition that they arrive with a sound mind, free of concussion injury. Asking to come out of the game due to a "bell ringer" should be endorsed and commonplace, with no guilt or shame attached.

Parents: Parents must prioritize the athlete's health and well-being higher than the outcome of the game or scholarship. Society does not expect our youth to have the knowledge or judgment to provide informed consent when it comes to accepting the risk of playing contact and collision sports. It falls upon the parents and guardians to educate themselves, evaluate the risks and benefits of playing sports before allowing their children to participate. Parents and guardians are the front line when it comes to passing this information on to their kids, emphasizing prevention, sportsmanlike conduct, and prioritizing brain health over gameplay not only for themselves but their teammates. Parents need to know and recognize the symptoms of concussion injury because the athlete probably won't come home and tell them how they're feeling or about being hit. They also need to become familiar with the recovery protocols and expectations.

Coaches: Coaches need to support the culture change within the organization that embraces concussion awareness and management, and be able to recognize signs and symptoms. Typically, coaches will be the first ones to see the hit and resulting effects. Coaches have to put their winning records below the health and future of their players.

Athletic Directors: Being responsible for athletic programming, school athletic directors are responsible for the athletes, coaching staffs, trainers, school administrators, and medical personnel, assuring involvement in a clinical-caliber concussion management effort. Athletic directors should monitor its concussion protocols and invest in programs, tools, and personnel that serve the brain health of everyone involved in sports.

Athletic Trainers: When available, athletic trainers should be the first-line of defense with administering concussion management including concussion education, baseline measurement, sideline assessment, reporting and overseeing recovery care. Athletic trainers must be empowered to pull athletes from action if they suspect a concussion, and monitor the athlete's recovery progress, making recommendations for safe return to action and academic activities.

Referees: Although impartial to the outcome of the game, the referees should be partial to the health of the athletes, recognizing the severity of a hit and symptoms. Of course, they are also responsible to uphold the sportsmanlike conduct on the field and the safety rules of the game, being free to penalize for illegal hits to the head. I would like to give referees greater authority to pull players to the sideline if they suspect a concussion-like hit.

Medical Community: Unfortunately, too often Emergency Room and primary care providers will conclude after a CT scan the athlete is fine. But these scans do not rule out concussions and only help assess more serious injuries like skull fractures or presence of bleeding in or around the brain. The medical community needs appropriate concussion awareness and training of concussion-management methods to play an informed role in the health of the athlete.

School Staff: Academic performance can be an indicator of a concussed student-athlete. Teachers, counselors, and other academic administrators need to know the signs and symptoms, and understand the concussion may be impairing the student. Here again, the "invisible injury" is all too often minimized, and "return to learn" accommodations ignored, resulting in provocation of symptoms, longer recovery times, and injured athletes falling behind in their curriculums.

League Officials: From the NFL, NHL, and NCAA, league officials and conference directors are obligated to institute concussion-management programming at the highest level, to protect the athletes' future and themselves from future legal tangles. Additionally, rules of the game need to be continually monitored and enforced to ensure the safety of the athletes.

Team Owners: On the professional level, I would encourage ownership to invest in its athletes' futures, setting aside income for their futures off the field. This may involve encouraging athletes to retire early if brain trauma is suspected, and provide income that is invested in the players' future business and/or health needs. I believe player contracts should include terms related to brain health, adherence to brain health protocols, and rules.

White House Pitches In

The White House recently joined the concussion fray, hosting a "Safe Sports Concussion Summit" (May, 2014). President Obama announced several initiatives to research concussions, involving a number of organizations and millions of dollars. While research is important and helpful for the future, the President appeared more interested in obtaining positive press, than actually applying our current knowledge to develop solutions to the problem now.

Still, the White House concussion summit helped promote further awareness of the cultural challenge sports face—even President Obama admitted to it. A few days later, *The Boston Globe* published an editorial which also points to the need to change the sports culture, saying:

> *THE SINGLE most important thing President Obama said at his well-intentioned, but ultimately ineffectual summit on the concussion danger in sports last week was,* **"We have to change a culture that says you suck it up"** *... It is good for the president to add his voice to those concerned about head injuries. But young people still lace up for sports where the culture and risks of being hit in the head have barely changed. That means we are still telling them to suck it up.*

Pride is a Problem

In February 2014, leading up to the NFL Super Bowl between the Seattle Seahawks and Denver Broncos, I was involved with the #C4CT

Concussion Summit at the United Nations building in New York City. Numerous scientists presented their latest findings regarding concussion, which was all very interesting. But the most compelling information came from active and retired players themselves.

- ***Clinton Portis***, former NFL running back said during the Concussion Summit that getting hit hard and getting back up is a matter of pride for players.

  "The pride of being a running back was having pride in colliding with the other guy and hitting them as hard or harder than they hit you," Portis said. "But you don't realize how hard you were hit."

  He is feeling the effects now. "I had a memory that was so crisp and now it's not as crisp as it was. My vision used to be one of my strengths, now it's not and I'm having migraines," said Portis, who played nine seasons in the NFL.

- ***E. J. Henderson***, a former NFL player, said he never had a medical diagnosis of a concussion, but during the game all players "remember those hits" that cause temporary concern. "Now I notice memory loss and a short-temper and I've only been out of the game for two years."

- ***Robert Griffith*** played 13 seasons in the NFL said his job playing strong safety was to be an "enforcer." In one game, Griffith said he told himself "we are killing each other out here." Griffith said NFL players are often looked at as "heroes," but people need to realize concussions are making them "damaged goods." "I think we all (former NFL players) have some short-term memory issues. I have to keep notes of everything and have my phone with me all the time," he said. "I now know the affects of the game because after four or five years, I began to see problems among players with sleep, depression, addiction, self-worth, and mood swings."

- ***Lance Johnstone***, played in the NFL for 11 seasons only missing nine games. He was also never medically diagnosed with a concussion. "But I can't tell you how many times I had to close one eye to see straight," Johnstone said. "As a player, you start to accept new norms of pain. Now I'm 40-years-old and I'm scared honestly. I have brain fogginess, a memory that things just slip my mind, and really have to concentrate in order to focus."

- *Isaiah Kacyvenski*, who is a former seven-year linebacker in the NFL, said players become experts at playing with or hiding pain. "The men who make it all the way to the NFL must become masters at masking pain," he said. "I never wanted to speak up about any issue I felt, particularly about concussions because they are known as 'unknown risks.'" After football, Kacyvenski earned an MBA from Harvard Business School, a seemingly impossible accomplishment after years of hard hits to the head. "Losing focus is one of the most frustrating experiences," Kacyvenski said about his studying years. "I had to battle to get through school. Was I different after football? Unequivocally, YES."

- *Percy Harvin*, offensive standout for NFL Champions Seattle Seahawks, sustained a hard hit in a playoff game a few weeks earlier against the New Orleans Saints. He walked off the field showing signs of concussion. "I was dazed, but wanted to come back," Harvin said during the Super Bowl Media Day about that hit. "I was saying to myself 'how could this happen?'" Harvin had just returned after an 11-game recovery from a hip injury. But somehow, Harvin passed the sideline concussion assessment and was allowed back into the game. Within a few plays, he sustained another blow to the head. This time, the concussion symptoms were more evident and he missed the rest of the game, and the following NFC Championship game against the 49ers.

ESPN Football Analyst, John Clayton, said during Super Bowl week the biggest challenge with concussions is "players are always going to want to get back on the field as soon as possible." The toughness culture nurtures players' pride about their ability to sustain hard hits. It's this nature that is killing brain cells causing cognitive and emotional impairment and even lives. Clayton said even though scientists are studying concussions, and helmet manufacturers are advancing their protection, most people don't realize that all it takes is a hard fall to the ground. "One dimension that rarely gets covered is the recoil effect on the brain," Clayton said. "It happens all the time, every game someone has one." However, not everyone reports concussion symptoms because of the toughness mindset.

"The NFL needs stronger protocols for how they handle it," Clayton said speaking of hard falls, hits, and the machismo preventing players from reporting concussions.

Obviously professional athletes have millions of dollars of earning potential at risk with reporting concussions. The pride of being able to sustain and deliver blows is a cultural phenomenon that's not helping the problem.

It's time to redefine toughness in the game. While I believe mental and physical toughness to endure hardship are great assets, the brain physiology cannot cooperate. Perhaps we will see a new era in sports where toughness means having the humility to admit your brain is more important than the game.

Should We Take the Helmets OFF?

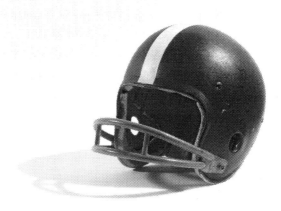

At the White House, "Safe Sports Concussion Summit," President Obama announced that concussions are now a national priority. He said more research is needed, more awareness, better protocols, and better equipment. What if safety equipment was contributing to the problem?

As absurd as this may sound, research suggests that this is a serious issue. American football players don their gear before hitting the fields like gladiators of the Roman Empire or the Knights of the Round Table. Of course, the intent to require such gear for gameplay is to protect the athlete as much as possible from injury due to contact or collision. Yet, an unexpected phenomenon occurs. The athlete, particularly the youth athlete, now has a sense of invincibility. The athlete now is more likely to engage in risky behavior because of a confidence that the gear will protect him from injury. Even worse, the athlete may now feel "weaponized" to the point where he will intentionally use his armored body and head as a missile to inflict injury.

An athlete once told me that one of the immediate goals of the game is to inflict pain on the opponent. "Hit them hard enough that it hurts and they will be slow to get up, and think twice about entering your territory," he said. "You feel bad if you've caused an injury, so you want to hurt them but not break them."

How does the athlete know what kind of force he is delivering to his opponent? With this weaponized self perception, how can he judge what kind of collision will injure and what will "just hurt."

The equipment designed to protect our athletes may, in fact, be weaponizing them and decreasing their sense of vulnerability.

This phenomenon is known as *"risk compensation,"* a psychological concept, which suggests that people adjust their behavior in response to the perceived level of risk, becoming more careful when they sense greater risk and less careful if they feel more protected.

Translation
If you wear safety equipment, you're inclined to take greater risk.

The theory emerged after several road-safety interventions failed to meet expectations and perhaps had the opposite effect. This "Peltzman Effect," named after Sam Peltzman, a professor of economics at the University of Chicago Booth School of Business, was reported in 1975 with controversy. Peltzman's study suggested increased highway safety regulation did not decrease highway deaths, saying "regulation was at best useless, at worst counterproductive."

More studies ensued in other applications, including:

- Cyclists wearing helmets rode faster, <u>Risk Analysis</u>, 2011.
- Drivers drive faster, less carefully wearing seat belts, <u>Accident Analysis and Prevention</u>, 1994.
- Condoms seem to foster disinhibition, <u>The Lancet</u>, 2009.

Safety Equipment Helping or Hindering?

Football equipment has come a long way since it's rugby-like days in late 1860s, when some players strapped crude leather "head harnesses" around their head. Around 1905, mounting concerns about serious injuries occurring led many colleges to ban the game altogether. Then, President Theodore Roosevelt stepped in to help save the newly-loved game, forming what would become the National Collegiate Athletic Association (NCAA).

In the 1939, the NCAA required helmets, which the National Football League (NFL) followed suit in 1943, to reduce the risk of injury.

Today's American football players wear "Iron Man-like" armor, galvanized head to toe with thick synthetic materials. The shoulder pads stack 4 to 6 inches high, capable of absorbing—and delivering—enormous force. Helmets surround the skull snugly, protecting the skin and skull with virtually unbreakable polycarbonate alloy plastic, but surprisingly do little to protect the brain inside. Chest vests, appearing bullet-proof, cover the abdomen with extra protection.

Today's athletes are bigger, stronger, faster and have become finely-tuned collision machines capable of producing greater force than ever.

Would they hurl themselves with such abandon if they did not wear all the safety equipment, like rugby players?

Lesson from Rugby

While rugby and American football have evolved from a common past, the games have many differences including rules and equipment designed to protect the athletes.

According to Jim McKenna, a professor at Leeds Metropolitan University (and a rugby coach), American football players often tackle head first which is seldom seen in rugby. "Their head is the tip of the missile, with an enormous body of weight behind them," says McKenna. Meanwhile, the helmets and padding can actually make the situation worse, he thinks, encouraging them to use more force.

Maybe there's a safety lesson we can derive from rugby? Dr. Warren King, a team doctor for the Oakland Raiders and who has also worked with the U.S. National Rugby team thinks so.

"I think the biggest thing football can learn from rugby is that, no, you can't use the head as a weapon," Dr. King said.

Rugby's contact rules are centered around the wrap tackle. A tackler can't slam into the ball carrier. He has to wrap his arms around and bring him to the ground. Tackling around the neck or head is illegal. Tackling low—around the ankles or knees—is fine, but because you have to wrap up, you're not barreling into a player, which leads to various injuries.

Without helmets (although some rugby players wear padded hats that are a little like football helmets from the 1920s), rugby players are taught from an early age to get their head to the side and make contact with the shoulder.

Dr. King added that helmets are a double-edged sword as they can give an athlete a false sense of security (risk compensation) and risk of repetitive concussions remains despite the latest technology.

"We're learning more and more that these small concussions over time in a variety of sports can have a serious, lasting effect later in life," Dr. King said.

Safety gear may dull the impact to the body, but no equipment can dull the impact to the brain. No matter how much protection you add, there's no such thing as a "concussion-proof helmet." The brain was not meant to sustain the force caused by athletes crashing headfirst into each other while wearing helmets and padding designed to absorb impact. Ironically, this equipment may put athletes' futures at greater risk.

It's a radical thought, but what if the game of football was to ban helmets altogether? John Tamny, reporting for *Forbes* agrees, writing in 2012 that "if so, players will be far more careful about how they hit and tackle, and they'll do both with much less force."

Since the game itself has become more of a violent spectacle than athletic prowess, here are a few ideas to avoid risk compensation injury.

Tips to Avoid Risk Compensation Injury

1. Educate parents, coaches, and athletes about the risk compensation phenomena. Safety gear is for protection, and does not make athletes invincible or allow them to take more risks or be more aggressive.
2. Teach proper, alternative tackling techniques, in football.
3. Add non-contact practices to focus on strategy, technique instead of hitting.
4. Increase enforcement of rules, or alter them, to reflect desire to protect athletes from brain injury. Add penalties as necessary.
5. Promote significant penalties for any "bounty" that encourages gladiator attitude to hurt an opponent.

The only way to intervene is by proper instruction and role modeling by coaches and parents, and proper enforcement of the rules of the game that are meant to protect the players from injury.

Concussion Laws Changing Culture

Starting the process toward a cultural shift in sports, in the last few years, every state in the United States has enacted student-athlete concussion laws that require sports programs offered at high schools and colleges to provide elements of concussion management. Inspired by Zack Lystedt, a former high schooler who nearly died on the field after he suffered a concussion and continued playing, Washington D.C. called it's concussion legislation the "Lystedt Law."

While each state differs a bit in what they require, most include moderate forms of education and protection,[8] including:

- Requiring parents or guardians to sign a concussion-information form.
- Removing student-athletes suspected of concussions from play.
- Making concussed student-athletes obtain medical clearance before returning.

Complying with these laws has started to impact the culture that may be causing concussions. But I fear many parents, coaches, and athletes treat compliance as another red-tape inconvenience. Although it's a start, these laws lack luster, adequate monitoring, and most have no penalty for non-compliance. For example:

- Requiring parents to sign a concussion-information form or "consent-form," doesn't serve as adequate education, in my opinion.
- Removing suspected concussed athletes from play, doesn't address detection standards or return-to-play guidelines.
- Obtaining medical clearance prior to allowing a concussed athlete to return to play, assumes the medical professional is well versed in concussions and related brain trauma.

Therefore, I'd recommend states begin amending their first stab at student-athlete concussion laws to include:

- Educational activity that verifies the individuals demonstrate understanding of the material, e.g., passing a test. Society expects such demonstration of skill and knowledge to safely operate a car or boat, why not do the same to safely playing sports?
- Adding concussion awareness responsibility beyond parents, coaches, and athletes to include team medical professionals, academic teachers, referees and, of course, athletic trainers, athletic directors, and league officials.

---

[8] A state-by-state listing of these student-athlete concussion laws can be found at edweek.org and searching the site for "Concussion Laws By State."

- Concussion detection should be standardized to some degree, so we all are using compliant tools and technologies.
- Return-to-Learn guidelines should be included as well, protecting student-athletes from certain school activities that may delay the healing process.
- Medical personnel, specifically trained in concussions, should give Return-to-Play clearance.
- Pre-season baseline testing should be required for all athletes. I believe this should be given as often as pre-season physical exams—regardless of the sport.
- The concussion laws should reach beyond schools, and into club levels, and other non-school sponsored youth leagues.
- Penalties should be established to add teeth for lack of compliance. Therefore, these laws need to be monitored, and when they are not followed, the proper authorities should be enabled to penalize accordingly.

The brain is the single most important organ to provide a long, healthy life. And, participating in sports can provide healthy development for an individual's development, personality, physique, and overall self-esteem and identity. Therefore, a paradigm shift needs to occur with contact sports organizations that emphasizes brain health as much as X's and O's. We need to be much more mindful about our players minds. After all, doesn't everyone desire a peak performing brain that can execute quickly, accurately, effectively, on and off the field?

Cultural Change Examples

I envision an era when contact sports and concussion management are discussed simultaneously, throughout the teams' preparation. Here are some examples:

- Pre-season concussion education for everyone involved in the student-athletes' development.
- Pre-season baseline testing for all athletes, recorded, and monitored throughout the player's career.

- Tackling techniques should be taught to avoid direct-head contact.
- Rules designed to protect the head, should be taught and enforced to a greater degree.
- Concussion assessment should occur virtually anytime an athlete shows problems with understanding material, confusion, vacant stares ("spacing out"), headaches, and slow responsiveness. A concussion-caliber hit may have occurred, but was not noticed so these symptoms give team leadership "just cause" to require a concussion test.

With my protocol, I've taken concussion management to a level never seen before in sports. It exceeds necessary compliance with state laws, even the NFL's protocol, providing guidance throughout the season. *See* Chapter 8 for details to my program.

Status of Current Concussion Management

The phrase "concussion management" is a relatively new concept in sports, which refers to the system, protocol, or plan for managing concussions. Regardless of the age, sport or level, a program should be in place to handle all aspects of the concussion —from education, baseline testing, sideline assessments, reporting, daily symptom tracking, and recovery care guidance.

Previous eras in sport would basically ignore hits to the head, sweeping them under the rug with off-base suggestions to "walk it off." In the last 10 years or so, tools have been made available to help measure concussion risks, but could hardly be considered "concussion management" programs.

More recently, largely due to the enormous media attention given to concussions resulting from NFL lawsuits and former NFL player suicides, a renewed emphasis on how to manage concussions has evolved. At best, we are still in an "early-adopter" phase of concussion management, but I envision within the next five years, concussion management will become as relevant as the sport itself.

The current status of concussion management depends on the level of participation. The professional levels have the most resources, so they have fairly sound methods and personnel to manage concussions with multiple athletes and varying degrees of severity. College and high schools will typically have athletic trainers, who have some education about detection, prevention, and protection. Youth leagues and clubs rely heavily on coaches, parents, and volunteers to help with injuries and concussions, with varying—if not minimal—levels of education.

In light of such disparity in concussion education and management protocols, many companies have rushed to develop tools and methods to assist. However, they too vary widely, which give all sports programs a significant challenge to protect the most important asset on the team— their players' brains.

The challenge is this, how does a program—with athletic trainers or not—educate all involved parties effectively; record baseline measures with cognitive, balance, and emotional categories; detect possible risks from the sideline or locker room; provide effective reporting to responsible individuals; track symptoms daily; and provide guidance to the recovery process?

Athletic Trainers Leading the Way

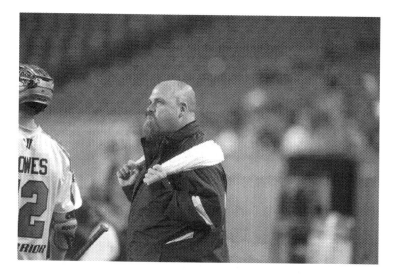

Across the nation, sports organizations are wrestling with this dilemma that's not going to go away. Perhaps on the forefront of concussion management are the athletic trainers serving on the high school and collegiate levels.

Athletic trainers are required to have bachelor's degrees with studies in nutrition, exercise physiology, kinesiology, and biomechanics. Most programs want athletic trainers with master's degrees, accreditation, or certification in various athletic training education.

The regarded National Athletic Training Association (NATA) defines athletic trainers as healthcare professionals who recognize, prevent, and rehabilitate injuries that result from playing sports or other physical activities. They may be part of a complete health care team and work under a physician's supervision. Athletic trainers provide medical and allied health care services to individual athletes or entire sports teams. Elementary or high schools, colleges, and professional sports organizations, as well as medical centers may employ them.

However, there is limited concussion and brain-related education course work required. Most athletic trainers must seek out concussion education because the topic is obviously important, relevant to their work, and increasing in prevalence.

Athletic trainers must also sort through various tests, tools, and techniques to assemble their own makeshift concussion protocol and make necessary recommendations to upper level management regarding in which to invest. Most opt for just having a baseline test, comply with state concussion laws, and add on additional education as fast as possible by providing a "concussion sheet" that must be signed by athlete and parent.

When an athletic trainer, who may be responsible for the health of hundreds of athletes at a time, has multiple concussions to manage, varying levels of severity, and recovery timelines, just managing concussion injuries alone can create a major life and death challenge.

In the absence of an athletic trainer, when a concussion occurs, a trip to the emergency room often ensues. The ER doctors, although well-versed in a wide range of conditions and treatments, are not typically concussion specialists and will call for a CT scan. The CT scan does not reveal a concussion, but only bleeding, contusions, skull fractures, or obvious brain abnormalities. So, the athlete, diagnosed with concussion, is sent home to "take it easy" for a few days with minimal instructions as what to do or expect next and almost no information on the necessary steps required to return to normal activity and gameplay.

Helmet Hit Tracking Technology

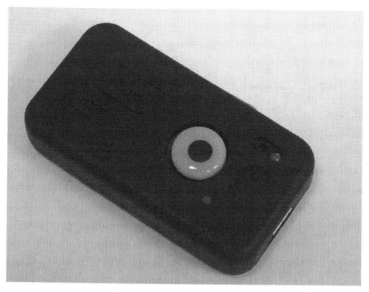

(Source: GforceTracker.com)

Tracking hits and measuring impact velocity are new ways to count hits much like baseball pitchers count their pitches. The theory says that the more hits a player sustains, the more risk the player is to long-term consequences of repetitive brain trauma. Adding accelerometers and sensors to helmets help provide data, and I believe this technology should be pursued. I also believe helmet safety enhancements should continue to be investigated. This technology cannot stand alone. It must be linked to the clinical picture. For instance, if a player sustains a 100g hit on the field, he or she may be required to come off the field for a sideline assessment using a standardized tool. If there are no signs of concussion, the athlete may be cleared by a medical professional to return to the game with close observation for the rest of that day and perhaps even the next few days. Like the pitch count, an athlete sustaining a number of sub-concussive hits—let's say at 20g, within a month or a season—may need to repeat their baseline computerized cognitive testing to make sure that these hits have not resulted in impairment of brain performance. However, while these sensors and technologies continue to develop, they still do not address the concussion management problem NOW.

There is a real void of tangible, measurable, and effective concussion management today, leaving sports programs in a vacant stare, much like the one they are trying to avoid.

Therefore, a grass-roots swell of activists, coalitions, books, and documentaries have emerged to help bring awareness, research, and programming to help. But inconclusive science, a variety of unregulated safety equipment, and lack of user-friendly and effective technology has created a real need for a fully-integrated, comprehensive, clinical-caliber program that anyone can use.

In the next chapter, I'll lay out the concussion management keys, introduce the concepts and tools integrated into my protocol, providing the basis for "Concussionology: Redefining Sports Concussion Management."

CHAPTER 8

CONCUSSIONOLOGY

Advancing Best Practices in Sports Concussion Management

For the majority of sports teams around the world, when a player exhibits signs of wooziness—a non-medical term for a legitimate symptom of a concussion—it's too late.

The player returns to the team huddle, masking their rapid onset of brain fog by trying to be alert. Parents passionately scramble to the sidelines, hoping the best, fearing the worst. Well-meaning coaches keep the team focused on the short-term objective of winning the game. In the absence of an athletic trainer, teammate, or referee who recognizes the problem and has the fortitude to suggest the player take a timeout, the player engages in action without realizing the enormous risk they are taking.

Amidst conflicts of interest, player pride, lack of education, and a proper concussion management system in place, the risk of concussion and resulting possibility of long-lasting brain damage, leaves more questions than answers.

- How serious was the hit?
- Does the player often show these signs?
- Should you let the player continue playing?
- Should anyone do something?
- How do you tell if it's a concussion?

- If it is a concussion, then what?
- Has the player ever had a concussion before?
- Who needs to know?
- What should the concussed player do?
- What programs, tools, and tests should we administer?
- And the most common question is: When can the player return-to-play, or return-to-learn?

Not all concussions are alike. Some are obvious, others are not. If an athletic trainer is available, they must do their best to assess the injury in a timely manner.

The answers to these questions are not always straightforward. Managing concussions goes beyond diagnosing a concussion, which entails knowing the mechanism of injury, understanding signs and symptoms, conducting several clinical tests, and comparing them to baseline scores.

Despite the life-altering consequences that concussions can create, most sports teams manage concussions with one arm tied behind their back. Limited education, a dizzying array, and lack of clinical-caliber tools and systems have put concussion management in a gray area.

In this chapter, I'll review some "best practices" and keys to recommendations for a thorough concussion management protocol. Additionally, I'll introduce a comprehensive sports concussion management program that benefits from my personal experience and expertise treating hundreds, if not thousands, of concussions in my practice.

"Best Practices" Missing Links

A number of organizations have established guidelines, position statements or otherwise referred to as best practices, for managing concussions, including the following[9]:

- American Academy of Pediatrics (AAP)
- American Association of Neurology (AAN)
- American College of Sports Medicine (ACSM)

---

[9]   NOTE: The published Guidelines are available online.

- International Conference on Concussion in Sport
- National Athletic Trainers Association (NATA)
- National Collegiate Association of America (NCAA)

Currently, there is limited consensus across all these organizations regarding details in application. There is a convergence of opinion and they all include the following general outline:

- Education regarding concussion dangers, assessment, and recovery
- Pre-season baseline testing establishing a benchmark for cognitive performance, symptom inventories, and perhaps postural or balance tests
- Concussion assessment modalities during the season to address initial concussion risk and severity
- Post-concussion recovery care
- Medical clearance requirements for "return-to-play"

The missing link with all of the "best practices," is a fully integrated, end-to-end tool that can be used with any sport—any level that is practical, and relies on the evidence-based guidelines these respected organizations have provided. In other words, the theories need help with actual application in the current environment. The term "fully-integrated" refers to one system that seamlessly integrates all the necessary components including education, baseline testing, balance testing, sideline assessment, tools, post-injury assessment, monitoring, and recovery guidance. And, "end-to-end" refers to the ability to apply this program from the pre-season preparation all the way through to returning the athlete to normal activity and gameplay. Of course, this data and technology could also follow the athlete throughout this career and lifetime.

Soon after the State of Maryland passed mandatory concussion management protocols for youth athletes, the local school district in my area approached me with a dilemma. The state had defined mandatory requirements for public schools to have written concussion management programs, policies, and procedures and mandatory concussion awareness education and return-to-play protocols requiring medical professional clearance for youth athletes, yet left the local districts on their own to develop them. My school district neither had the knowledge nor the means to develop such a program, so the school administrators reached out to me for assistance. As we developed the local district's program, it was readily apparent that the most efficient method of meeting the state's requirements, was to make the program entirely Internet based. The connectivity of the Internet, mobile applications' capabilities on smartphones, and advances with database integration, could be leveraged into a single tool, accessible anywhere, anytime. The days of holding up two fingers, asking how many do they see, penciling in checkmarks on a score sheet, entering data into a spreadsheet, and tracking players injuries by Rolodex® cards had come to an end.

XLNTbrain offers a complete feature set when compared to other solutions.

	NFL Protocol	ImPACT Test	Concussion Vital Signs	XLNTbrain
Downloadable and fully customizable Policies and Procedures Document				✓
State Legislation Compliant Online Educational Activity				✓
Online Baseline Testing	✓	✓	✓	✓
Preseason compliance tracking and reporting				✓
Mobile Sideline Assessment Tool				✓
Mobile Balance Test				✓
Concussion incident reporting		✓		✓
Email alerts with notification and post-concussion instructions going to athletes, parents, and healthcare providers upon concussion reporting				✓
Symptom checklist reporting and tracking				✓
Concussion Recovery Tracker with 5 Step Progressive Exertion				✓
Academic Care Plan generation based on symptoms				✓

When developing my protocol, I reviewed virtually all the position statements and guidelines available, so my system would meet or exceed the published recommendations. I wanted to raise the bar on concussion management and establish a new standard of care. I found the best practices were not embracing the technological age or neurological intelligence. My conclusion is the sports world is starving for a seamless, thorough and practical sports concussion management solution that is simplified with technology.

For example:

- Internet-based computer technology offers a centralized method of accomplishing each of the steps in the concussion management process, integrating all the data into a single source in real-time.
- Video training delivered online educates proper concussion awareness for athletes, parents, coaches and educators to optimize prevention, recognize the presence of concussion related symptoms and encourage a cultural shift towards prioritizing brain health over gameplay. Including a short quiz after watching the training, verifies the individual has watched and comprehended the material. This educational activity can be monitored by supervisors who can then identify who has, and has not completed the training. This far exceeds most state concussion laws that merely require the athlete, parent and team athletic trainers to sign off on a form.
- Smartphone technology is now at a level of sophistication to integrate assessment tools to assist responsible adults at the sidelines to document potential concussion incidents. This technology also allows injured players a convenient method of documenting concussion-related symptoms during the post-concussion recovery phase.
- The immediate connectivity of the Internet and email allows for instant alerts of potential concussion events to all key individuals involved in the athlete care. Athletic trainers and other healthcare providers can track injured athletes' recovery progress in real-time, making post concussion management as efficient as possible. Reporting takes on other forms as well in a fully-integrated program. School administrators can instantly access data related

to athletes and parents completion of state mandated preseason activities, policies and procedures, and status of concussed athletes program wide.

- A fully-integrated, computer-based system also allows for the objectivity and transparency needed to manage concussion properly under the watchful eyes of league officials, union administrators and state regulators.
- Research applications abound for using a comprehensive, fully-integrated computerized concussion management system. Potential applications include evaluation of potential bio-markers to the vulnerability to concussion or the development of delayed effects of multiple brain trauma, clinical correlation of concussion incidence and severity to bio-mechanical measures such as accelerometer technology, and the effects of therapeutic interventions on outcome measures such as recovery time and cognitive performance.

A complete concussion management program that utilizes technology gives the sports world a chance to have a "virtual neurologist" on its team, ultimately preserving the athletes' health and optimizing their game performance.

The Four Rs

Rather than try to explain every best-practice guideline, differences, and programs available on the market, I've simplified the entire sports concussion management discussion into four categories, or "The Four Rs:"

Recognize

Provide proper awareness about how to recognize and recover from concussions, the potential short- and long-term impairments that complies with state laws. Recognize athletes' current condition with pre-season baseline testing that measures the full spectrum of cognitive and emotional performance tasks.

Report

Gain the ability to immediately assess, document and report results of concussion symptoms to necessary parties including the athlete, parents, coaching and training staff, athletic trainers and athletic directors, medical professionals, and if necessary, league officials.

Recovery

Guide the athlete and training staff through a progressive exertion protocol that helps determine when the athlete can be cleared to "Return-to-Play," as well as "Return-to-Learn" academic activities.

Responsibility

It takes a "team effort" to apply concussion management involving the athlete, parents, coach, training staff, medical professionals, referees, league officials. The health of the athlete's short- and long-term future should weigh heavier than the desire to return to the field or the classroom.

Taking a closer look at each of the Four Rs, let's outline my concussion management protocol.

Note: Every sports team should enlist a "concussion coordinator," typically an athletic trainer if available, who administers and monitors the concussion management throughout the season. This individual will be responsible for each of the "Four Rs," administering, monitoring and reporting progress at any step.

Recognize

There are two steps to "recognize" concussions in this protocol, including *education and baseline testing,* both of which occur prior to the pre-season. It's also advisable to recognize the *gender differences* that may influence pre-season baseline scores.

Education

Every state in the U.S. requires high school and youth sports teams using public facilities and their coaches to receive a certain amount of concussion awareness education every year. The education must, obviously, comply with state-wide regulations about causes, symptoms of concussion, potential short and longterm consequences of concussion injury, and importance of correct concussion treatment.

Athletic trainers, and other medical professionals who deal with concussions, should obtain annual concussion education, because the field is emerging with new studies and practices that would enable to adapt their care based on the latest science.

However, the education activity typically used by school systems and youth organizations is little more than reading and signing a consent form. I believe the education activity must involve verification the individual has showed an adequate level of comprehension, thus requiring a quiz be taken after receiving the education training.

Through my protocol, participants receive thorough training, articles and blogs about concussions and the latest news reports about the emerging concussion management topic. Upon subscription, the user—or concussion coordinator—may administer the concussion video training, or the participants may view the program online from a computer with internet access. After the individual(s) reviews the training video, an interactive quiz must be taken to complete the educational activity. This pass-fail score is recorded, enabling the concussion coordinator to track and report the team's participation.

In the absence of my all-inclusive system, the concussion coordinator must select adequate concussion education and organize a method of administering the education, showing comprehension of the material, as well as monitor and report participation.

Baseline Testing

Many concussions can be managed without post-injury cognitive testing, however post-injury testing can be indispensable. The problem is that one can never predict which athlete will benefit from having baseline testing performed. So, when possible, every athlete should take a "baseline" test prior to the season, establishing normal cognitive and emotional measures for future comparison. Baseline testing is critical to measuring cognitive changes due to traumatic injury. Baseline tests, which vary considerably, typically take about 20-40 minutes to complete, measuring an athlete's memory, attention and concentration, problem solving abilities, and processing speed down to the millisecond. From this testing, we are able to determine the level of functioning prior to any brain injury, and compare the results with those taken after a concussion is suspected during the season. The level of variance between the pre-season baseline and the post injury tests can help measure the severity of the concussion, provide objective measures of concussion-related impairment, what area of the brain may be suffering and what symptoms to begin tracking towards the recovery timeline.

Based on my experience, and listening to athletic trainers administering baseline tests, I found existing baseline tests to be cumbersome to interpret, and not necessarily efficient or comprehensive for the typical concussion coordinator's needs. Additionally, the majority of baseline tests are not integrated into a comprehensive, single platform to enable the management of the entire protocol. Therefore, I developed my own version, and incorporated it into my concussion management modality.

My Baseline Test is a web-based, neuro-cognitive test measuring:

- Baseline presence of concussion-like symptoms
- Reaction time
- Attention
- Inhibition
- Impulsivity
- Memory
- Information processing efficiency
- Executive function

The test also assesses emotional reactivity, mood, worry, and anger domains, major distinguishing factors from all other sports concussion tools currently on the market.

Upon completion, the results are then compared with a normative database of all these measures, giving the concussion coordinator and medical professionals insight with establishing level of risk each athlete may have going into the season. These results also establish a baseline score to compare with later should a concussion injury occur.

Gender Differences

I recently studied over 1,300 high school and collegiate athletes, ages 14 to 22, to examine the possibility of gender differences among pre-season concussion symptoms. Using my Sport Concussion Symptom Checklist, we asked each participant to score themselves in seven domains including cognitive, vestibular (dizziness, balance, coordination), sleep, migraine, mood, worry, and anger.

Analysis of the seven symptom complex domains demonstrated statistically significant increased symptom scores for female athletes in the following domains: vestibular, sleep, worry, migraine, and mood domains. No difference was found in the cognitive or anger domains. Age-related differences were not found.

Said more simply, females are more likely to express their symptoms than males, who may experience the symptoms but not be willing to express them.

The conclusion is that significant gender differences exist in the endorsement (acknowledging and admitting experiencing the symptom) of concussion-related symptoms in high school and collegiate athletes at baseline; female athletes being more likely to endorse these symptoms with vestibular, sleep, worry, and mood domains. These gender differences should be taken into account when assessing athletes for concussion-related symptoms.

The concussion coordinator and medical professionals need to be aware of these differences between men and women, recognizing males are less likely to express all their symptoms during the pre-season baseline test and after injury.

In the absence of my program, a concussion coordinator must develop the baseline testing program, administer the test to the athletes, interpret the results, take time to record the results and organize them for future reference, in order to demonstrate compliance with the concussion management program.

Report

When pre-season conditioning and practice begins, the concussion coordinator should be equipped to detect, record, and report concussions, or suspected concussions, to all involved parties. Easy to say in one sentence, but more difficult to accomplish.

Armed with knowledge of concussion risks and symptoms and the pre-season baseline test results, the concussion coordinator must have a few more items to be easily accessible during practice and games:

- Names and contact information for the athletes, including parents, coaches, athletic trainers, and medical professionals (see "Responsibility" below) among others.
- Concussion detection protocols or modalities to be applied during practice or game play. These are often referred to as "sideline assessments tools."
- Access to email or phone to report suspected risk of concussion, and begin the recovery process.
- As an added layer of protection for contact and collision sports, I also recommend equipping the athletes with impact sensors, such as GForceTracker, Inc. (GFT). These Hit Count Certified (by the Sports Legacy Institute) impact sensors track the number and force of hits sustained by the head, giving the concussion coordinator a valuable tool of identifying when an athlete may be at risk.

Several brands of head impact indicators are available that sense force and/or acceleration of impacts to the head. These devices are not meant to diagnose concussion, but rather to detect the frequency and magnitude of impacts to the head.

It is important to note that there is little evidence to suggest an impact threshold for a concussion exists. Each concussion is different and some may result from higher magnitude impacts, while others may occur at lower force levels. Still, impact sensors like GFT help establish a measurement standard for the number of hits and force of collision and rotation. What is of ultimate importance is to correlate the force of a single hit or a string of sub-concussive hits, with the presentation of symptoms or impairment of cognitive performance. I've included an article about "3 Ways to Integrate Impact Sensors Into Concussion Management Protocol", in the Appendix G.

Sideline Assessments

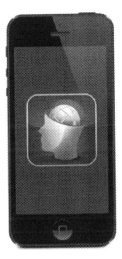

As practice begins, the concussion coordinator must be equipped with a tool, test, or device that guides the sideline assessment process of identifying risk of the presence of concussion.

In my work with concussed patients, I found a void between concussion assessments, baseline scores and reporting capabilities that was integrated into one tool. So, I created a Sideline Assessment Tool and Balance Test. Both of these deliver the convenience of documenting the condition of the athlete at the time of a possible concussion based via a mobile app available on smartphones. (A print-out version is also available.) After assessing a potential concussion on the sideline or in the locker room, the Sideline Assessment Tool automatically documents the findings and emails an alert to all-involved parties, including parents, team coaching and training staff, and medical professionals that a report has been filed.

Among other tools is the Sports Concussion Assessment Test-3 (SCAT3), which can be printed and available during practices and games. While the SCAT3 is helpful, it is not integrated into a comprehensive concussion management system.

Another concussion-assessment tool, King-Devick Test, measures oculomotor function, responsible for eyeball and eyelid movement. The test uses rapid number naming that involves reading a string of numbers on three test cards to measure for saccades, attention, concentration, speech, and language. Significantly slower times, indicate presence of concussion risk. While this assesses oculomotor function on the sideline as part of the concussion assessment battery, it also is not integrated into a comprehensive concussion management system, and it does not assess for other features of acute concussion injury such as balance, memory impairment, or disorientation.

Ultimately, the concussion assessment is critical to the concussion-management system, giving concussion coordinators the ability to perform a series of sideline assessments, describe the condition of the athlete, and assist in on-the-field decision making by medical professionals. Even when a medical professional is not available at the sideline, the sideline assessment is invaluable to the medical professional that will ultimately be responsible for the injured athlete, providing essential information regarding what the athlete looked like at the time of the injury.

The "X" factors are the athletes themselves, and time. A culture must be created that encourages athletes to report their own symptoms as accurately as possible. The athlete, coach, athletic trainer, and parents should be aware that often concussion symptoms appear hours or even days later. Therefore, if there is any hint of a concussion-related symptom, I suggest giving the sideline assessment after the athlete has had the chance to rest on the sideline, before making the return-to-play decision. "When in doubt, sit them out" is the mantra for sport-related concussion injury.

Recovery

My biggest concern is allowing an athlete suspected of having a concussion to "return-to-play," even to normal academic activities, too soon. While athletes may say they feel "fine," with the game on the line, too often they are put in harm's way by returning to action prior allowing the brain to heal. Even the "return-to-learn" decision should be calculated into the recovery process.

Recovery from a concussion can be an elusive process. Feeling "fine" does not always mean the brain is ready for another impact, and the injury itself maybe affecting the athlete's judgment and self assessment much in the same way as alcohol often impairs an individual's judgment about his ability to drive. In general, the brain and body need time to rest for a period of time. The amount of time varies from one individual to the next. During this recovery period, the injured athlete's symptoms need to be monitored. Before the athlete can resume gameplay, medical clearance must be given.

The recovery discussion is a bit of a gray area for most people, even medical professionals. So, I've integrated a process into my concussion protocol to provide the athlete and medical professionals data and guidance to assist with obtaining medical clearance.

Recovering from a concussion begins with "relative rest," minimizing mental and physical stimulation until the athlete is symptom free. *Relative rest* refers to the avoidance of any mental or physical activity that provokes the athlete's concussion-related symptoms.

Return-to-Learn

Resting the brain includes taking a break from typical academic activities. Healing from a concussion can be delayed if the athlete's brain is forced to memorize, focus, make decisions, endure test-taking stress as well as other anxieties. This is another gray area not addressed in most concussion management protocols—except in my protocol. Student-athletes are students first. The course of their recovery may include the need for an academic care plan of school accommodations that is customized to each individual injured athlete to allow the student to return to the academic environment while minimizing provocation of symptoms. Inspired by the most recent American Academy of Pediatrics guideline recommendations, my system automatically maps a concussed athlete's symptoms to the appropriate academic accommodations for the return-to-learn process.

Once the injured player is free of symptoms at rest, I have included a 5-Step Progressive Exertion recovery guide built in that monitors symptoms, and guides the timeline for return-to-practice and gameplay.

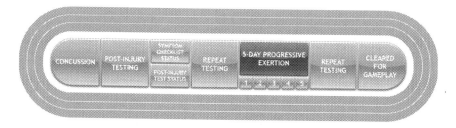

Within the my concussion management system is a Recovery protocol that begins when a concussion is suspected. It includes:

- Post-injury testing using the Sideline Assessment Tool and Balance Test.
- Daily symptom checklist tracking online or using the smartphone app, with immediate results and easy-to-read tracking for medical professionals.
- Post-injury test status, using the brain-cog test to compare to pre-injury performance.
- 5-Step Progressive Exertion plan with a series of stages of physical exertion while simultaneously monitoring symptoms on a daily basis and post injury brain-cog testing after full exertion to aid in return-to-play decision making.

Clearance for Gameplay

Armed with this data, a medical professional can review the progress, daily symptoms, scoring on all the tests, and make an informed decision.

The goal is to return the athlete back to action safely. The gradual progression of mental and physical activity, while monitoring cognitive performance and daily symptom checklists help athletes, parents, coaches, and medical professionals avoid the dangers associated with concussions and returning too early.

Responsibility

Compliance and applying complete concussion management involves a community team effort. There needs to be a cultural shift towards prioritizing brain health over gameplay that involves virtually everyone involved in the sport, starting with the athlete themselves (*see* Chapter 7).

Every athlete needs to take responsibility for his or her brain health. It's time for a paradigm shift to occur where athletes are more concerned about their futures than their performance on the field. This cultural shift requires others' support. As stated earlier, every team needs to have a "concussion coordinator" responsible for carrying out a complete "end-to-end" protocol throughout the season or school year.

My concussion protocol involves each individual responsible for the sport and athletes' care. Incorporating them from the beginning to the end of the season.

All-In-One Platform

Concussion coordinators, athletic trainers, and anyone else involved in preventing, detecting, and protecting athletes from concussions have a major challenge. Sports-related concussions are developing an emerging field with many existing and new tools available. I empathize this for those responsible for the athletes' concussion care and who do not have a single platform they utilize.

An affordable, multifaceted concussion management system, designed by a neurologist that is integrated into one system would simplify and enhance the level of care to new heights and become a new standard in the sports world.

My concussion management system was designed to accomplish this goal and equip sports teams with clinical-caliber guidance to recognize, report, and recover from concussions throughout the season. It's like having a "virtual neurologist" on your team.

CHAPTER 9

RE-BUILDING THE BRAIN

Reversing Damage Caused by Concussions

The brain's delicacy and vulnerability to damage from concussions and repeated sub-concussive hits, is also capable of healing. The brain may show signs of degeneration over time, it can also regenerate itself given the right environment.

Although most people rarely think about their brain health, the brain changes throughout life. During embryonic development and early life, the brain changes dramatically. Neurons form many new connections, and some neurons die. From early childhood to early adulthood, the brain continues to develop until around the age of 25-years-old. Even in the adult brain, neurons continue to form new connections, strengthen existing connections, or eliminate connections as we continue to learn. Recent studies have shown reversing brain damage caused from years of playing football is possible, and neurons have capability to regenerate if the conditions are right.

Unfortunately, most people don't realize it. Even sadder, some professional athletes have lost their lives because they didn't realize the changes in their brain could be rehabilitated.

Remember Junior Seau, NFL star linebacker? He was 43-years-old when he took his own life in May 2012. His brain was donated to science for research. The National Institute of Health (NIH) later found he suffered from *chronic traumatic encephalopathy* (CTE). As explained earlier, CTE is a degenerative brain condition caused by repeated head traumas like sub-concussive hits.

In April 2012, Atlanta Falcon safety Ray Easterling, at 62-years-old took his own life, and his autopsy found signs of CTE.

Then, there's Dave Duerson, former Chicago Bears defensive back, who at the age of 50, shot himself in the chest so his brain could be researched. It was, at Boston University, where they found CTE as well.

Jovan Belcher, NFL linebacker with a promising career in front of him, fatally shot his girlfriend before firing the gun on himself in 2013. These are only a few extreme examples among hundreds of other former NFL players troubled by brain trauma.

But you don't have to be a professional football player to struggle with brain health. Regardless of your sport, your age, and your level of competition, the brain was not designed to sustain significant impact caused by blunt force.

However, there is hope. It's perhaps the most exciting discovery in medicine today. We can rehabilitate the brain. You don't have to donate your brain for research. We already know, can diagnose, and provide treatment to avoid making disastrous decisions, while rehabilitating the brain performance.

In this chapter, I'll outline keys to healing from a concussion during the first 30 days. Then, I'll share some scientific discoveries about reversing brain damage, and include a foundational principles for rebuilding the brain due to concussion, and long-term changes to the physiology of the brain resulting from repeated hits to the head.

Post-Concussion Treatment: Healing from Concussion During First 30 Days

Immediately after a concussion occurs, the brain begins the healing process. Over the course of next few days and up to about 30 days, it's critical to accept my treatment strategy and do…

Nothing

The brain physiology, blood flow and neuronal pathways all need to rest. Particularly the first 24 to 72 hours, I recommend minimizing any activity that provokes the symptoms of concussion. This includes physical and mental stimulation that may interrupt the healing process by forcing the brain to work. I use the phrase "brain sprain" because like an ankle sprain, you have to limit movement so the muscles, tendons, and ligaments get a chance to return to normal before adding any more pressure to the wound.

During the *acute phase*, meaning the period of time immediately following a concussion injury, the brain requires rest while dealing with the metabolic demands of repairing the affected brain cell membranes which have been stretched. PET scan studies show that *glucose*, the primary energy source, is not able to freely get into the brain cells as usual, preventing the cell's ability to get the fuel to supply the demand for repair or proper functioning into the cell. In other words, the damaged brain cells are grasping for energy, but they cannot get the fuel.

Thus, the need for rest, as well as healthy foods, plenty of water, and perhaps nutritional supplements are needed to support the healing process.

Within a day or two of the concussion, while symptomatically at rest, don't jog, run, lift weights, or do any kind of physical exercise because it pumps more blood into the "leaky" brain cells that are trying to heal. Also, avoid any mental activity like reading, writing, texting, learning, even talking. Avoid the sunlight or well-lit rooms when sensitive, because the eyes and nervous system pathways that take in visual stimuli may also be affected. Even watching movies, playing video games, loud music, working on the computer, or trying to fix something may all exasperate the concussion healing. The brain is involved with everything we do, so for the first day or two, just rest.

When the initial symptoms have dissipated, that doesn't mean the concussion has healed and the athlete is ready for action or the classroom. Now, we move into a phase I refer to as "relative rest," minimizing mental and physical stimulation until the athlete is symptom free during activity. *Relative rest* refers to gradually liberalizing mental or physical activity, still avoiding those that provoke the athlete's concussion-related symptoms.

As mentioned earlier, once the injured player is free of symptoms at rest, I begin a 5-Step Progressive Exertion recovery guide, which is built into my platform that monitors symptoms and guides the timeline for a return-to-practice and gameplay.

During this recovery phase, each day presents tasks with increased levels of difficulty. Should any of the concussion symptoms reappear, then it's back one day, to the previous level of activity, which did not provoke symptoms.

However, if the athlete progresses each day through recovery without provoking any symptoms, then the brain is healing from the trauma. When the athlete can complete all the "5-Steps" of the Progressive Exertion plan and their cognitive performance remains at baseline, then they can seek medical permission to return-to-play.

Typically, this allows for a seven-day cycle. But it could vary, and I'd recommend erring on the side of caution, without rushing the return to normal activity and gameplay.

One of the reasons recovery time can vary is because athletes with a history of previous concussions may require longer periods of time to heal. A study reported in *Neurosurgery* in 2007, indicated the presence of long-term residual visual-motor disintegration in concussed individuals with normal neuropsychological measures. Most importantly, athletes with a history of previous concussion demonstrate significantly slower rates of recovery of neurological functions after the second episode of mTBI.

Many other factors influence the concussion recovery time in addition to previous history of concussion like the severity of the concussion, level of pain, and personal lifestyle factors such as history of drug abuse, alcohol use, exposure to toxic environments, previous brain-related impairments, even genetic history. Every brain is different, every brain injury varies. Most healthy athletes, however, will see significant improvement within 7 to 10 days following their concussion, with 93 to 97% recovered by day 30.

Relieving Pain

In the first 24 hours after sustaining a concussion, the person should not take any pain medications. A pain medication can "mask" the symptoms, which could allow someone to return to activities with a concussion. As stated, many concussion symptoms will take several minutes, hours, or days to arise. After this 24-hour period, should the athlete experience a severe headache, I recommend taking an anti-inflammatory, over the counter, *acetaminophen.* Naproxen, aspirin, and ibuprofen (NSAID-type medications) should not be used at first, as they may increase the risk of bleeding. Beyond this, ask your doctor for help with addressing any other pain.

Sleep

Insomnia is a common post injury symptom. I recommend a temporary sleep aid. Over the counter remedies are usually made of antihistamines which are sedating for most people and help improve sleep quality. However, it is not uncommon for some people to become more alert with antihistamines worsening the insomnia. Short-term use of traditional sleep aids is appropriate in this setting. A doctor may even recommend taking *imipramine,* a tricyclic antidepressant, which not only helps with sleep but also can help protect against headaches and improve cognitive performance.

Post-Concussion Recovery Recap

Post-concussion symptoms typically last about 7 to 10 days, depending on how severe the concussion is and other factors. Most people get better within a week, however, that varies based on how well they adhere to the recovery protocol.

General advice for treating a concussion includes the following:

Sleep: Contrary to some common belief, sleep is the first and best thing to do to help recover from a concussion. Try to get at least 7 to 8 hours of sleep per night within the first week of sustaining a concussion.

Mental Rest: The brain needs to rest while recovering. Avoid strenuous mental activities during the first few days after sustaining a concussion to avoid provoking symptoms. Limit reading, writing, texting, using computer, and playing video games. Also avoid other visual and auditory stimulus like bright lights and loud music.

Physical Rest: Engage in no physical exercise until symptom free. Exercise adds strain on the brain, delaying the healing process.

Eat Healthy: The brain needs a nutritional diet and perhaps some nutritional supplements, such as Omega 3 fatty acids, Vitamin B Complex, Vitamin E, CoQ10, and other brain healthy supplements to enhance the healing process.

Drink Water: The brain needs water to facilitate returning to proper balance. Aim for 100 oz. per day.

Additional Advice

- Avoid toxins, such as drinking alcohol, and smoking.
- Ease into normal activities slowly, not all at once. Follow my Recovery Protocol for guidance about when to return to the sport or school.
- Make sure to let employers or teachers know that you had a concussion.
- Avoid activities that could lead to another concussion, not only sports, but also certain amusement park rides, or (for children) playground activities.
- Avoid driving, operating machinery, or riding a bike (since a concussion can slow one's reflexes).
- If necessary, discuss with your employer or professors if it is possible to return to work gradually (for example, starting with half-days at first). Students may need to spend fewer hours at school, have frequent rest periods, or more time to complete tests.
- Take only those drugs approved by your doctor.

- For some people, an airplane flight shortly after a concussion can make symptoms worse.
- After completing the 5-Step Progressive Exertion protocol and the athlete is symptom-free, retake the baseline test, and see your doctor to obtain clearance to return to gameplay and the classroom.

Frequently Asked Questions

What if the head injury happens during a game or sport?

- An injured athlete should come out of the game or practice immediately to be tested on the sidelines by a person trained in concussion assessment, and using a quality test or toolset like my Sideline Assessment Tool. An athlete with concussion symptoms should not play again that day, and should not play as long as symptoms are present. The athlete might need to wait 1 to 2 weeks or longer before being cleared to play again.
- The concussion coordinator, coaches, and trainers can help the treatment process by noting the following information:
    - The cause of the injury
    - The force of the blow to the head or body, which may include an impact sensor
    - Loss of consciousness and for how long
    - Any memory loss following the injury
    - Any seizures following the injury
    - Number of previous concussions (if any)

When should an athlete with a possible concussion go to the emergency room?

- A loss of consciousness (greater than one minute), a neck injury, or symptoms such as weakness or numbness, double vision that persist, and worsening of condition, severe (incapacitating) headache, or "something is just not right," are reasons to send the athlete to the emergency room.

When can an athlete return to play after a concussion?

- Before an athlete can return to play, he or she must be totally symptom-free and return to his or her baseline (pre-concussion) scores. Once the athlete has returned to baseline, he or she should start a five-day program in which he or she increases activities while any symptoms are monitored. If any symptoms return, the athlete should return to the previous level of asymptomatic activity. My recovery protocol includes a Daily Symptom Tracking tool, and 5-Step Progressive Exertion plan.
- While recovering from a concussion, it is important to avoid anything that could cause another jolt or blow to the head or body. *Once you have a concussion, you are at three to five times greater risk for later concussions.* A repeat concussion that occurs before the brain has recovered from a first one can slow permanent recovery and increase the chances for long-lasting problems. These problems include difficulties with concentration and memory, headaches, and sometimes physical skills such as keeping one's balance.

What pain medications can be taken for a concussion?

- In the first phase of concussion, the person should not take any pain medications. A pain medication can "mask" the symptoms, which could alert medical personnel to the presence of a more serious injury.
- After a concussion is diagnosed, acetaminophen can be used; however, it should not be given just to cover up headaches. Naproxen, aspirin, and ibuprofen (NSAID-type medications) should not be used at first, as they may increase the risk of bleeding.

What are the risks of suffering permanent brain damage after having a concussion?

- The level of risk of sustaining permanent brain damage depends on the individual's brain health, and history of previous concussions and sub-concussive hits. Typically, having one concussion will not lead to long-term impairments. The primary risk of long-term brain damage occurs when a second concussion is sustained while a previous concussion is healing. This is known as Second-Impact Syndrome.
- Additionally, a damaged brain will likely degenerate faster with age, leading to increased risk of early onset of Alzheimer's disease, dementia, memory loss, depression and a host of other cognitive and emotional impairments.

Danger Signs — Adults

In rare cases, along with a concussion, a dangerous blood clot may form on the brain and crowd the brain against the skull. Contact your doctor or emergency room right away if, after a blow or jolt to the head, you have any of these danger signs:

- Headaches that are incapacitating or get worse in the first 24 hours
- Weakness, numbness, or decreased coordination
- Repeated vomiting
- Lethargy or cannot be awakened
- Have one pupil—the black part in the middle of the eye—larger than the other
- Experience convulsions or seizures
- Have slurred speech
- Experience persistent double vision
- Are getting more and more confused, restless, or agitated
- Distinct personality changes, e.g., unnecessary anger or emotional outbursts
- Trouble with decision making
- Persistent confusion and getting lost

Danger Signs — Children

Take your child to the emergency clinic right away if they show these signs:

- Has any of the danger signs for adults (see above)
- Won't stop crying
- Can't be consoled
- Won't eat

Although you should contact your child's doctor if your child vomits more than once or twice, vomiting is more common in younger children and is less likely to be an urgent sign of danger than it is in an adult.

Rehabbing Brain Drain: Addressing Sustained Symptoms Beyond 30 Days

Typically, healing from a concussion and restoring equilibrium within the brain's cell membranes usually takes 6 to 10 days, and can be as short as one day, or as long as a month. However, should symptoms resulting from a concussion continue beyond 30 days, the brain may be suffering from a more significant injury to the tissue and changes to the brain physiology that require more than rest and "relative rest."

This opens the door to the new frontier in science, and perhaps some of the most exciting discoveries in medicine, showing rehabilitating the brain from various trauma is not only possible but likely, given the right treatment. However, the opposite is also true—a damaged brain will likely degenerate faster with age, leading to increased risk of early onset of Alzheimer's disease, dementia, memory loss, depression and a host of other cognitive and emotional impairments (*see* Chapter 6 on "Brain Drama").

Along with me at the forefront of studying ways to reverse brain damage is Daniel Amen, M.D., founder and CEO of Amen Clinics, Inc., and two-time board-certified psychiatrist. He led three groundbreaking clinical studies of 135 active and former players from the National Football

League using brain SPECT imaging (single photon emission computed tomography) to measure before and after results.

"Our studies found significant evidence that, fortunately, there are treatment protocols that can often reverse many of the symptoms caused by brain damage and improve brain function," said Dr. Amen.

Here's a snapshot of three published studies that I believe show significant evidence of brain damage caused by football, and that related brain performance can be improved. Working with more than 100 or more active and retired professional football players, Dr. Amen continues to lead the largest brain-imaging study ever conducted.

"Impact of Playing Professional American Football on Long Term Brain Function"
published in the *Journal of Neuropsychiatry and Clinical Neurosciences*
Winter 2011

Abstract Brief: This is the first large-scale brain-imaging study to demonstrate significant differences consistent with a chronic brain trauma pattern in professional football players.

"Effects of Elevated Body Mass in Professional American Football Players on rCBF and Cognitive Function"
published in *Translational Psychiatry*
2012

Abstract Brief: The study showed overweight NFL players with brain damage from repetitive concussions might be at heightened risk for cognitive impairment. Moreover, overweight athletes had significant decrease in attention, general cognitive proficiency, and memory. These findings suggest that a weight management program may be critical to the health of athletes who have been exposed to mild brain trauma during their careers.

Perhaps one of the most exciting studies conducted by Dr. Amen showed brain-damaged NFL players improved their cognitive performance after a clinical intervention that included lifestyle changes. Below is the study for your reference:

"Reversing Brain Damage in Former NFL Players: Implications for TBI and Substance Abuse Rehabilitation"
published in the *Journal of Psychoactive Drugs*
2011

Abstract Brief: An open label pragmatic clinical and lifestyle intervention was conducted with retired NFL players who demonstrated brain damage and cognitive impairment. After six months of complying with the intervention methods, the athletes showed statistically significant increases in attention, memory, reasoning, information processing speed and accuracy. Many athletes had greater than 50% increases in percentile scores.

The findings should have significant impact on the football and medical community, as well as anyone with brain damage due to concussions, chronic traumatic encephalopathy (CTE), toxicity from alcohol and drug use, and other brain traumas. It's encouraging news for anyone, at any age, that it's possible to reverse brain damage.

Re-Building the Brain

Based on the studies above, we can surmise that playing professional football is potentially bad for your brain; people with history of concussions, who are also overweight, have decreased brain performance; and that, brain function can be improved. So, the next logical question is, how can we rebuild the brain?

I typically look at the following domains of brain-related performance:

- Cognitive (thinking, memory, decision making, focus, attention)
- Migraine
- Vestibular (balance, posture, spacial orientation)
- Sleep (sleeplessness, over sleeping)
- Mood

- Worry
- Anger

Now, we'll look at several modalities and treatment options designed to enhance brain performance in each of the domains listed above.

Neurofeedback

One tool that can benefit all of the domains, except vestibular, is neurofeedback. Neurofeedback is a type of biofeedback that measures brain waves in real-time to produce a signal that can be used as feedback on brain activity to teach self-regulation—or re-training the brain. Neurofeedback is commonly provided using video or sound, with positive feedback—or a reward system—for desired or optimal brain activity. It can be guided by qEEG (quantitative EEG analysis) that is usually used in clinical settings.

The analysis is displayed on a computer, as the brain goes in and out of inefficient states. The technique detects when the brain is in a more stable state, when that happens the computer will generate a reward—like a bell, a point in a game, an animation that moves —a variety of reward systems can be used. The principle is: Reward the brain, and the brain will naturally spend more time in the rewarded state. It's a form of physiological manipulation of the neurons in the brain.

Neurofeedback treatments typically begin at one 30-minute session per week for 3-6 weeks. The number of session vary according to the quality of the technology applied. For example, with newer technology, you can apply 18 to 20 sensors on the brain, and train numerous structures and networks simultaneously. So the more advanced the technology, the more efficient and lower number of visits will be necessary. With neurofeedback, you can also target specific areas of the brain where there has been trauma, like from a concussion.

The emotional trauma associated with athletes who have sustained head injury, can develop a difficult to diagnose but serious condition called post-traumatic stress disorder (PTSD). PTSD can show up in a variety of ways. Symptoms may include flashbacks, nightmares, and severe anxiety, as well as uncontrollable thoughts about the traumatic event. PTSD can lead to many troubling cognitive, emotional, and behavioral problems.

I've also found a neurofeedback intervention to be an excellent tool to manage PTSD.[10]

Migraine Intervention

The most common symptom that plagues many people with prior concussion or other brain trauma is recurrent migraine headaches. Occurring more often in women than men, migraines can be debilitating due to the pain. After 30 days of receiving a concussion, if headache pain escalates, then medical intervention may be recommended.

The migraine can progress through four stages, though not all people experience all the stages, including:

Prodome: One or two days prior to the migraine, you may experience symptoms that signal a oncoming migraine such as: constipation, depression, food cravings, hyperactivity, irritability, neck stiffness, uncontrollable yawning.

Aura: A nervous system disturbance prior to or during a migraine that may include visual phenomena (flashes of light, seeing various shapes, bright spots) or sensory (feeling pins and needles in arm or leg), verbal (speech or language problems) and temporary vision loss.

Attack: The migraine attack may last 4 to 72 hours, but frequency varies. Symptoms include pulsating or throbbing pain on one or both sides of the head, sensitivity to light, sounds or smells, nausea, blurred vision, and lightheadedness and sometime fainting.

Postdrome: After an attack, you may feel drained and washed out, while other people report feeling mildly euphoric.

---

[10] **Note:** Neurofeedback is relatively affordable, depending on your location and availability to the treatment. Typically, neurofeedback is administered by psychologists.

Should migraines persist beyond 30 days after the concussion, and over-the-counter medication does not relieve the symptoms, see your doctor who may prescribe one of the following:

- Triptans — Primarily prescribed for acute relief of mid-level pain and not considered a cure. Triptans include sumatriptan from the family of tryptamine-based drugs.
- Topiramate — An anticonvulsant originally used to treat epilepsy. It is also FDA-approved for the prevention of migraines.
- Valproic Acid — Approved by the FDA for the prevention of migraines, Valproic Acid helps prevent migraines by restoring balance of the physiology of the brain.
- *Imipramine* — Helps prevent migraine pain, improve sleep, and treats post-concussive syndrome.
- *Propranolol* — A beta-blocker that treats high blood pressure, anxiety, and panic; also prevents migraines.

These examples of medications can help reduce the frequency and severity of migraines or stop the migraine process once it has started. If treatment isn't working, talk to your doctor about trying a different migraine headache medication. The right medicines, combined with self-help remedies, and lifestyle changes, may make a big difference.[11]

Fueling Memory

One long-term consequence that some people have after suffering brain trauma such as a concussion, is related to cognitive function and memory loss. Short-term memory lapses, in particular, may be a sign the brain is not receiving enough fuel to function. The brain depends on *glucose* as the main energy source for its physiological and pathological function, including keeping neurotransmitters at peak levels.

---

[11] **Please note:** This information is provided to educate readers on health care and related medical conditions but it is not intended to be a recommendation or to replace the guidance of a licensed physician.

If glucose is lacking, neurotransmitters are not synthesized and communication between neurons break down. Age also plays a role in glucose utilization since an older brain uses more glucose than a younger one to perform the same learning and memory tasks.

Abnormally low levels of one neurotransmitter, called *acetylcholine,* has been found in people with *Alzheimer's disease* which is a degenerative disorder affecting memory.

One possible explanation for the brain's reduced ability of some areas to metabolize glucose is when the brain cell's membranes have stretched to the point they are unable to regulate the presence of glucose. Glucose does not easily pass through the cell membrane on its own. It requires the help of a glucose transporter protein. It is postulated that the glucose transporter protein is not functioning properly in certain diseases such as Alzheimer's. This dysfunction may explain why PET scans, after acute concussion injury, also show low neuronal glucose uptake, in spite of the increased metabolic demand needed for healing and restoration of equilibrium. This is the energy crisis of concussion injury. Therefore, if you can fuel the brain with an alternate source that bypasses the need for glucose, you may be able to restore brain function.

One treatment for Alzheimer's, approved by the FDA, is a medical food called *Axona (caprylic acid)* that provides the brain an alternate fuel source. Axona is a form of medium-chain fatty acids (MCFA), deriving typically from palm or coconut oils, which the body can transform into *ketones.* The brain can utilize ketones as a source of energy, supplying up to two-thirds of what's needed, bypassing the need for glucose while targeting the metabolic deficit.

Making Memories

While providing the brain more fuel to function properly, there are a variety of ways to improve your memory. Generally, memory comes in three forms:

- *Working memory* or residing in the frontal lobes provides the ability to pay attention and may last less than a minute.
- *Short-term memory* from inside the temporal lobes called the hippocampus recalls details from the last few minutes to a few weeks which are deemed necessary or novel.

- *Long-term memory* on events, details, relationships that are able to be recalled from many years back are most likely due to a series of synapses that involve many areas of the brain and related senses. Science still doesn't have a pure understanding of how long-term memory works.

We do know the brain can create new cells and pathways. Like a muscle, exercising the brain's memory functions can improve your working short- and long-term memory. Also, like a muscle, the brain's memory capability can weaken if it gets bored and is not challenged, like going into "auto-pilot" when driving home on the same route.

So the key to exercising your memory muscle is to provide it new challenges, new learnings, new skills particularly if it involves multiple areas of the brain like movement, and the five senses including visual, auditory, smell, taste, and touch. A few excellent examples include:

- *Get Your Groove On* — Learning a new dance challenges the brain to work in several different ways, including coordinating movement with music, sequence of steps, processing visual cues, speaking the steps and then adding your own creativity to the dance while practicing all give the brain's memory a healthy workout.
- *Habla usted Espanol?* — Learning a new language, and its affiliated culture, helps the brain's memory-functioning and auditory-processing, even with learning sign language. Additionally, taking in the culinary, societal, and historical differences about a cultural gives the brain great exercise and ability to learn new things.
- *Play That Tune* — Learning to play a new instrument, learning to sing a new song, or even writing a new song all tap the brain to exercise it's memory with auditory signals, visual cues, and lyric memorization.
- *Pre-game Preparation* — Athletes may be more inclined to exercise their memory with helpful information to enhance their performance. Scouting the opposition, identifying players' strengths

and weakness, observing and writing down the opponent's plays and sets are all helpful. Also, athletes that learn new skills, new techniques, new strategies in game situations, and learning new plays all serve to exercise your brain's memory muscle.

- *The Power of the Pen* — While there are many tricks to memorization, which we won't get into here, another tool to help build memory capability is to break out a pen and paper and do some writing. Whether you write about your thoughts and experiences, stories, poetry, or write down important information you want to remember, connections get built in the brain when you think, form a sentence, write it down so you can see it, hear it, and feel it.

Brain Gym Training

The brain controls everything we do and every body function, whether we realize it or not. So, the brain needs more than memory-building exercises. Rehabilitating the brain that has suffered from a concussion or repeated hits to the head, may require exercising other areas of the brain due to multiple issues affecting its cognitive performance.

For example, functions related to forethought, judgment, decision-making, and planning are served by the prefrontal cortex (front, forehead), which is a common damaged area among athletes, particularly football players. Or perhaps the temporal lobes (on right and left sides) may have been affected by trauma. These are emotional centers that may need some new connections.

All the other areas of the brain (*see* Chapter 3) can benefit from frequent and regular trips to the "brain gym," whether it's a hi-tech online brain training service, or a low-tech strategy.

Hi-Tech: *Virtual brain gyms*, a variety of computerized online brain training tools, are available. Of course, it requires access to a computer with an Internet connection. The best brain gyms will be guided through a self-assessment that measures and identifies your brain's strengths and weaknesses and then provides correlating exercises to train those specific areas. At-a-glance, you may interpret the brain exercises as glorified "video games," but they serve a purpose that combines neurology and technology to improve your brain's functions. These exercises are helpful, not hurtful like many commercial video games that over stimulate and dull the senses and remorse for death and destruction.

Low-Tech: *Brain teasing* games are simple crossword puzzles, word-finding games, Scrabble™, and other word games and puzzles which give the brain a workout. Learning and playing Chess is an excellent game for developing forethought, decision-making, and strategy. But you can also benefit from going to the local library or educational store and picking up some elementary or high school workbooks with various forms of topics, reading, and writing exercises, which is great stimulation for the brain.

Don't Snooze Past This

The human brain and body require rest, whether they are injured or not. Sleep doesn't get the attention it deserves, until you wake up after a poor night's sleep feeling groggy and having slow reaction times, clouded judgment, blurry vision, and a bad attitude—all signs of a tired brain. String a few days in a row with lack of sleep and you feel more like a monster than a human being.

The damaged brain relies on sleep to restore balance during the healing process. A lack of enough quality sleep can lead to a host of physiological and psychological problems, even dangerous consequences if you feel fatigue while behind the wheel.

- The National Sleep Foundation estimates 71,000 injuries and 5,500 deaths occur per year due to drivers who reported being drowsy.

The brain and body is a miraculous machine, but adults over the age of 19 must have 7 to 8 hours of sleep per night in order for them to perform properly. The younger you are, the more sleep is required. Consider this:

Average Sleep Requirements By Age[12]

Age (in years)	Hours of Sleep (in hours)
1–3	12–14
2–5	11–13
5–12	10–11
13–19	9
19+	7–8

Sleep also leads to peak athletic performance, according to researchers at Stanford University, who studied the relationship between sleep and athletic performance on six basketball players and men and women swim team members. The study measured speed and skills after normal night's sleep and after having extra sleep. Both their skills' accuracy and speed were increased after having extra sleep.

For those coming off a concussion and other brain trauma, sleep is a high priority. Sleep deprivation has been linked to a higher risk of depression, anxiety, ADD, Alzheimer's, Parkinson's, and other psychosis.

A variety of environmental, lifestyle, hormonal, and chemical-related reasons can be blamed on sleep struggles. But the main point here is, learn to get to sleep and stay asleep at all costs, especially when recovering from a concussion or post-concussion injury.

Here are a few tips:

- Make sleep a priority. Sleep shouldn't be the last thing you think about at the end of the day. Instead, create a bedtime routine that winds down your thoughts and actions to prepare for sleep. For example, take a warm bath or shower, do some deep breathing exercises, keep lights low, turn off the TV, and maybe read something light, encouraging or motivational.

---

[12] Source: National Sleep Foundation, National Institute of Neurological Disorders and Stroke

- Avoid anything that stimulates your senses within an hour of bedtime, e.g., loud music, bright lights, scary movies.
- Don't eat or drink caffeine and alcohol for two to three hours before going to bed.
- Add soothing sounds around bedtime to signal the brain it's time to rest, e.g., nature sounds like ocean waves, soft music, wind chimes, or even a fan.
- Use over-the-counter sleep aids sparingly. But they serve a purpose, as recommended by a doctor.
- Natural supplements can help nurture healthy sleep, including L-tryptophan, 5-HTP, valerian, kava kava, and melatonin.

If sleep continues to be a problem, see your doctor or sleep specialist who may want to conduct further tests to rule out other conditions that affect sleep. Prescription medicine exists to help with sleep, but be sure to get guidance from your doctor.

Food for Thought

Recommending a healthy, nutritious diet may seem like a doctor's default answer for everything. The latest scientific research shows the critical role nutrition plays in brain performance. Particularly for people with a history of brain trauma, like concussions or repeated sub-concussive hits, "you are what you eat," is a more accurate mantra than ever believed before.

While medications may intervene, reduce pain, and provide temporary solutions, utilizing nutrition as a natural alternative may be the key to healing brain trauma. Plus, as seen by Dr. Amen's study of NFL players with pre-existing history of brain trauma, being overweight reduces cognitive performance. So, getting your body weight in line with your age and height will give your brain a boost as well.

Overall, eating in a brain-healthy manner is simple, but for many it's easier said than done. Here is your guideline, in priority:

- Eat more vegetables than protein.
- Drink 100 ounces of water per day.

- Keep fruit to one or two servings a day.
- Eat complex carbohydrates like a side dish and avoid simple carbohydrates.

If you keep to these parameters, your brain and body will receive optimal nutrition ideally suited to support the energy requirements for the day.

It's easy to make excuses for eating food lacking in nutrition. Our society has created all kinds of processed foods, sweeteners, preservatives, soft drinks, snacks, and ways to deliver empty calories that do nothing but tell the body to store fat due to lack of nutrition. I would guess nearly 80 percent of people in America have these guidelines in reverse, for example:

- Eat excess bread, pasta, cereal, and rice.
- Protein dominates every meal. Vegetables are a side dish.
- Too much fruit, or none at all.
- Drink more coffee, soft drinks, and alcohol than water.

Every year a new diet and weight loss book gains popularity, and consumers eat them up. For the brain, my guidelines above serve as a simple principle: Fuel the brain with food, not fiction. Fictitious foods are manufactured, not harvested. If you can't pronounce the ingredient list, then the package contains fiction.

Ultimately, the body is designed to breakdown food into chemicals so they can be properly deployed, stored, or eliminated.

The Truth about Fats

The brain's solid weight is 60% fat, so we have to address fat when discussing re-building the brain. There are bad fats, called saturated fats and trans fats that you want to limit or avoid altogether. Saturated fats contribute to hardening of the arteries and plaque formation, which can block blood flow to the heart and brain. A 2009 study from British researchers found a diet high in saturated fats may lead to short-term memory loss and low energy. Saturated fats are derived from natural sources like red meat, egg yolks, and dairy foods.

More harmful than natural fats, are the man-made, chemically-altered trans fats. On labels, you can recognize these with terms like "partially hydrogenated" oils.

The good fats are called unsaturated and come in two varieties, monounsaturated and polyunsaturated *fat*. These fats actually help the body and brain function because they contain essential fatty acids (EFAs), called omega-3 fatty acids. They are "essential" because the body requires them and cannot manufacture them on its own. Omega-3 fatty acids are the gold gems of fats, and very important for recovering from brain damage.

While you can get omega-3 from eating fish and other plant-based sources like chia seed, perhaps the best source for omega-3 fatty acids comes from krill oil.

Krill oil is a unique source of omega-3 essential fatty acids extracted from Antarctic krill. These small, zooplankton crustaceans are at the base of the marine food chain, and the largest animal biomass in the world, weighing in at approximately 600 million tons.

Krill are rich in the omega-3 oils EPA (eicosapentaenoic acid) and DHA (docosahexaenoic acid), as well as phospholipids, flavonoids, and the carotene astaxanthin. The EPA and DHA in krill oil are incorporated into phospholipid molecules closely resembling that of brain phospholipids. This helps krill oil surpass fish oil because it's highly absorbable and bioavailable, as these essential fatty acids do not have to be converted in the body into cell membrane-ready phospholipids. The phospholipid form is both fat-soluble and water-soluble. In fish oil, the DHA and EPA are bonded to triglycerides, which is fat-soluble only. This difference has broad implications for digestibility, absorption, and utilization. Not to mention, taking krill oil typically does not result in fishy burps and aftertaste related to digestion reflux.

The super antioxidant *astaxanthin* gives krill oil staying power. Fish oil, on the other hand can oxidize, spoiling its benefits and releasing free radicals in the body. And, krill do not accumulate as many potentially harmful toxins and heavy metals as other marine life higher in the food chain. Some studies have shown that krill oil is significantly more potent than fish oil. This means you may need far less of it than fish oil, as confirmed by a 2011 study published in the journal *Lipids*.

Krill is also sustainable and an environmentally friendly source of omega-3. Krill harvesting in the Antarctic is regulated by the Commission for the Conservation of Antarctic Marine Living Resources (CCAMLR). This organization oversees sustainable krill fishery and has forecasted no shortage of krill.

Dr. Rudi Moerck, a drug industry insider and expert on omega-3 fats said, "Nothing else that has come along in the last 10 years, and nothing that I know of in the entire nutraceutical business, is as good for human health as krill oil."

All other omega-3 fats are extremely perishable, easily damaged by oxygen, whether animal-based or plant-based. However, krill oil contains astaxanthin, which prevents oxidative damage. In tests performed by Dr. Moerck, krill oil remained undamaged after being exposed to a steady flow of oxygen for 190 hours. Fish oil, however, went rancid after just one hour.

Due to krill oil's phospholipid makeup, which allows the body to absorb nearly all the omega-3 molecules, you may only need one 500 mg capsule per day.

Fish oil typically contains more EPA and DHA than krill oil. So, it remains a good source of omega-3. However, be sure to verify the fish oil's freshness, store it in the refrigerator, and don't buy it if it's in a clear bottle. Any fish oil dated over a year has probably perished.

The Alpha of Omega-3

Omega-3 is linked with benefiting health in a variety of ways including lowering cholesterol (LDL), boost brain function, fight inflammation, and is linked to helping prevent heart disease, improve skin elasticity, reduce PMS symptoms, as well as pain and stiffness associated with arthritis.

Research indicates that omega-3 deficiency can increase risk for a number of major diseases, such as type-2 diabetes, cardiovascular disease, cancer, arthritis, and others—and may actually accelerate the aging process. Low levels of omega-3 fatty acids have been associated with brain-related dysfunction such as depression, anxiety, ADD, suicide, and increased risk of Alzheimer's disease and dementia. DHA is a main component of the brain's synapses, while EPA improves blood flow, which boosts overall brain function. After all, the solid weight of the brain is 60 percent fat, so getting healthy fats from omega-3 sources is critical for optimal functioning.

Boosting omega-3 fatty acids also helps with weight loss because increasing omega-3 intake has been found to decrease appetite, cravings, and reduce body fat.

The Best Drink

The brain makeup is also predominantly water. Anything that dehydrates the brain, like too much caffeine or alcohol, can decrease cognitive functioning. To rehab the brain, you will need to begin to prefer water over any other liquid. Water helps the brain and body in many ways and can't be over-emphasized. Shoot for drinking 100 ounces per day for optimal brain health.

Besides water, I would also recommend switching to drinking green tea instead of coffee. Green tea has been associated with lowering risk of Alzheimer's because of its bioactive compounds and antioxidant benefits. Among the many benefits of green tea, is the active ingredient caffeine, which is a known stimulant.

Green tea doesn't contain as much caffeine as coffee, but enough to benefit the brain and body. Caffeine blocks an inhibitory neurotransmitter called *Adenosine*. This way, it actually increases the firing of neurons and the concentration of neurotransmitters like dopamine and norepinephrine.

Caffeine has been intensively studied before and consistently leads to improvements in various aspects of brain function, including improved mood, vigilance, reaction time, and memory.

Green tea also contains the amino acid L-Theanine, which is able to cross the blood-brain barrier. L-Theanine increases the activity of the inhibitory neurotransmitter GABA, which has anti-anxiety effects. It also increases dopamine and the production of alpha waves in the brain.

Studies show that caffeine and L-Theanine can have synergistic effects. The combination of the two is particularly potent at improving brain function.

Because of the L-Theanine and the smaller dose of caffeine, green tea can provide more sustained energy than coffee.

Bottom Line: Green tea contains less caffeine than coffee, but enough to produce an effect. It also contains the amino acid, L-Theanine, which can work synergistically with caffeine to improve brain function.

Sugar: Good or Bad for the Brain?

Since the brain's primary energy source is glucose, or sugar, it would seem a diet high in sugar would be reasonable, however this is wrong. That's because the body breaks down all ingested foods to their molecular level where the elements can be used, including converting carbohydrates into glucose.

However, eating too much sugar overloads the system, acting like an addictive drug that triggers the release of dopamine—the pleasure neuron. Sugar causes a blood sugar levels to spike, and then crash, leaving you feeling tired, irritable, and foggy. So, it's easy to eat more sugar to try to maintain the elated feeling.

Overeating, poor memory formation, learning disorders, depression—all have been linked in recent research to the over-consumption of sugar. These linkages point to a problem that is only beginning to be better understood—what our chronic intake of added sugar is doing to our brains.

A study published in *Neuroscience,* showed "a high-fat, refined sugar diet reduces hippocampal brain-derived neurotrophic factor, neuronal plasticity, and learning." In other words, a diet high in added sugar reduces the production of a brain chemical known as *brain-derived neurotrophic factor* (BDNF). Without BDNF, our brains can't form new memories and we can't learn (or remember) much of anything. Levels of BDNF are particularly low in people with an impaired glucose metabolism—diabetics and pre-diabetics—and as the amount of BDNF decreases, sugar metabolism worsens.

Chronically eating added sugar reduces BDNF, and then the lowered levels of the brain chemical begin contributing to insulin resistance, which leads to type-2 diabetes and metabolic syndrome, which eventually leads to a host of other health problems. Once that happens, your brain and body are in a destructive cycle that's difficult if not impossible to reverse.

Eating "added sugar," offers zero nutritional value and is called an "empty calorie," which the body stores as fat to be used for future use. This is the kind of fat stored around your belly and thighs.

So avoiding sugary treats, simple carbs, and anything labeled with "high fructose corn syrup" will benefit rehabbing a damaged brain. So instead of sugars, satisfy your sweet tooth with the natural sweetener called stevia.

Exercising the Body, Good for the Brain

Many athletes who trained at a high level may be susceptible to being overweight, because muscle can turn to fat. In the absence of regular training, practicing, and supervised strength and conditioning, athletes can go on an extended exercise holiday with unfortunate results. Being overweight can reduce the brain's effectiveness.

Physical exercise boosts brain functioning in a number ways and is perhaps the single most important strategy to enhance brain performance.

When you exercise, blood gets pumped throughout the body, which increases blood flow to the brain, supplying necessary oxygen, glucose, and nutrients to the brain. This activity helps grow new brain cells by boosting *BDFN*, a chemical that plays a role in neurogenesis.

Numerous studies shows exercise benefits learning as well. In 2005, *Pediatrics* published the results of a large-scale review of 850 studies showing the effects of exercise on academic performance. The panel of 13 researchers concluded optimal academic performance followed students who engaged in daily one-hour or more moderate to vigorous exercise.

Exercise boosts your mood too and alleviates symptoms of depression better than taking an anti-depressant medication called "Zoloft," according one study. Exercise also calms worries, boosts energy, helps improve sleep, burns fat, and a host of other benefits.

To rehabilitate the brain, incorporate cardiovascular exercise, resistance or strength training, as well as activities that require coordination. Dancing, doing Yoga, playing table tennis, learning a martial art, are good examples of coordination training.

Even walking briskly for 20 minutes a day will benefit the brain. So, don't make excuses, just go take a hike. Your brain and body will thank you for it later.

Natural Supplements that Boost the Brain

In Dr. Amen's, *Reversing Brain Damage* study on brain-damaged NFL players, the players showed significant cognitive and emotional improvements when making lifestyle changes such as eating a brain-healthy diet, not smoking, not recreational drug use, limiting alcohol consumption, and having a physical exercise regimen. But they also were on a strict regimen of taking natural supplements.

The study involved taking omega-3 rich fish oil (5.6 grams a day); a high-potency multiple vitamin; and a formulated brain enhancement supplement that included *phosphatidyslerine* and nutrients to enhance blood flow (*ginkgo* and *vinpocetine*), *acetylcholine* (acetyl-l-carnitine and huperzine A) and antioxidant activity (*alpha-lipoic acid* and *n-acetyl-cysteine*).

Additionally, *B vitamins* support the functioning of the nervous system, helping the brain synthesize neurotransmitters that affect mood and thinking. B vitamins are involved in helping the formation of brain chemicals such as dopamine, epinephrine, and serotonin, says Ray Sahelian, M.D. and author of *Mind Boosters*. In fact, each B vitamin plays its own role in preserving brain function and mental acuity. Starting from folic acid (a B complex), which helps in the early brain development, these vitamins help in many aspects of metabolism. A few recent studies have shown a link between declines in memory and Alzheimer's disease in the elderly and inadequate levels of folic acid, vitamin B12, and vitamin B6.

Coenzyme Q10 may have a place in the treatment of some neurological diseases. A placebo-controlled clinical trial of coenzyme Q10 suggested that it can slow the rate of deterioration in patients with early-stage Parkinson disease. The consumption of up to 800 mg per day of coenzyme Q10 was well tolerated. The trial was funded by NIH and appeared in the Archives of *Neurology* in 2002.

A host of research continues to find natural sources (vitamins, minerals, and herbs) to benefit brain function. But please note that one of the concerns about taking supplements is a lack of quality control because the FDA does not regulate vitamin and mineral manufacturing. So, it's important to find quality, trustworthy sources.

How Does That Make You Feel?

Despite all these ways to re-build the brain, there is absolutely no shame in addressing cognitive, emotional, and behavioral challenges within the context of working with a licensed therapist, psychologist, or psychiatrist. Many times, symptoms associated with mood swings, anxiety, and depression are linked to memories and events that have shaped our perspective on life. With professional guidance, you can re-train your brain and rebuild your life.

## CHAPTER 10

CONCLUSION

Concussionology

The topic of "concussions" continues to get more and more attention, and rightly so. The dangers associated with brain trauma are significant. In my opinion, the science and management of sports concussions finds itself to be an emerging field of study. It lays between neurology and sports medicine, hence the name "Concussionology."

It's critical that awareness, understanding, and treatment of concussions expands to all ages, levels, and sports. Using my concussion management online and mobile system provides an ideal modality that virtually any sports team and organization can implement. With it, your team will comply with state laws, and have a fully-integrated, clinical-caliber tool that simplifies concussion management based on my own background and experience as a neurologist.

The brain is an amazing organ, and we should do all that we can to protect it so that we can enjoy a future filled with memories and possibilities. And when the brain has been damaged, we need to take corrective action to rebuild it.

I love contact sports, but not the culture that breeds brain damage. I hope this book convinces you that it's time to redefine sports concussion management for the sake of the game and all the participants who put their brain on the line.

#

CONCUSSION RESEARCH, OTHER REFERENCES

The references below are available online at <u>xlntbrain.com</u>.

ACSM's Team Physicians Consensus Statement on Concussion: <u>http://journals.lww.com/acsm-msse/Fulltext/2006/02000/</u> <u>Concussion__Mild_Traumatic_Brain_Injury__and_the.29.aspx</u>

American Medical Society for Sports Medicine position statement: concussion in sport, Kimberly G Harmon, Jonathan A Drezner, Matthew Gammons, Kevin M Guskiewicz, Mark Halstead, Stanley A Herring, Jeffrey S Kutcher, Andrea Pana, Margot Putukian, William O Roberts. Endorsed by the National Trainers' Athletic Association and the American College of Sports Medicine, Published by British Journal of Sports Medicine (2013), 47(1), 15–26 (<u>http://bjsm.bmj.com/content/47/1/15.full.</u> <u>pdf+html</u>)

Almost Half of Homeless Men Had Traumatic Brain Injuries, <u>http://</u> <u>www.sciencedaily.com/releases/2014/04/140425104714.htm</u>

Athletic Trainer: Education Requirements & Career Summary, <u>http://education-portal.com/articles/Athletic_Trainer_Educational_</u> <u>Requirements_and_Career_Summary_for_the_Field_of_Athletic_</u> <u>Training.html</u>

Blood Test Identifies Brain Damage from Concussion In Ice Hockey, http://www.sciencedaily.com/releases/2014/03/140314093652.htm

Brain and Spinal Cord Injury, http://www.brainandspinalcord.org/recovery-traumatic-brain-injury/index.html

Brain Changes Can Result from Participation In One Year of Contact Sports, Evidence Shows, http://www.sciencedaily.com/releases/2014/04/140408154105.htm

Brain Injury Association of America, http://www.biausa.org/about-brain-injury.htm

Change Your Brain, Change Your Body, by Daniel G. Amen, M.D., Harmony Books, an imprint of the Crown Publishing Group, a division of Random House, Inc., New York. Copyright © 2010

Concussion and Mild TBI, Centers for Disease Control and Prevention. Accessed 4/30/2012.

Concussions and Our Kids: America's Leading Expert on How to Protect Young Athletes and Keep Sports Safe, Dr. Robert Cantu and Mark Hyman. New York: Houghton Mifflin Harcourt Publishing Company (reprint edition: September 24, 2013), 2012.

Concussion Crisis Growing in Girls' Soccer, Kate Snow, Sarah Koch, Deirdre Cohen, and Jessica Hopper. Rock Center, NBC News. 9 May 2012 (http://rockcenter.nbcnews.com/ news/2012/05/09/11604307-concussion-crisis-growing-in-girls-soccer?lite).

Concussion Knowledge of Primary Care Doctors Falls Short, Study Says: Many pediatricians, family practice doctors, internists lack confidence in concussion management abilities. Lindsey Barton Straus, JD, Moms Team Study. October 25, 2011, 17:45 (http://www.momsteam.com/print/3976).

Concussion Laws by State, http://www.edweek.org/ew/section/ infographics/37concussion_map.html

Consensus Statement on Concussion In Sport: the 4th International Conference on Concussion in Sport held in Zurich, November 2012, http://bjsm.bmj.com/content/47/5/250.full.pdf+html

Consensus Statement on Concussion in Sport: 3rd International Conference on Concussion in Sport, Zurich, November 2008, file:/// Users/davidjahr/Downloads/44484-44270-1-PB.pdf

Differential Rate of Recovery In Athletes after First and Second Concussion Episodes, Neurosurgery. 2007 Aug;61(2):338-44; discussion 344, http://www.ncbi.nlm.nih.gov/pubmed/17762746

Effects of Elevated Body Mass in Professional American Football Players on rCBF and Cognitive Function, *Transl Psychiatry (2012) 2, eK, doi:10.1038/tp.2011.67*

Epidemiology of Concussions Among United States High School Athletes in 20 Sports, Mallika Marar, Natalie M. McIlvain, BS, Sarah K. Fields, JD, PhD, and R. Dawn Comstock, PhD. The American Journal of Sports Medicine, April 2012. 40:747–755 (http://ajs.sagepub.com/ content/40/4/747).

Further Evidence of Link Between Concussion and Alzheimer's Disease, http://www.thefutureofhealthnow.com/concussions/, http://www.neurology.org/content/early/2013/12/26/01. wnl.0000438229.56094.54.short

Guidelines for Concussion Management in the School Setting, New York State Education Department, 2012, http://www.p12.nysed.gov/sss/ schoolhealth/ConcussionManageGuidelines.pdf

Head Injury as Risk Factor for Psychiatric Disorders, http://www.ncbi. nlm.nih.gov/pubmed/24322397

Head Injuries Can Make Children Loners, http://www.sciencedaily.com/releases/2014/04/140410083505.htm

Head Injuries Triple Long Term Risk of Early Death, Oxford University

Head trauma can cause chronic fatigue syndrome and fibromylgia, http://www.endfatigue.com/web-newsletters/Newsletter_3_head_trauma_cfs_fm.html

High School Concussions in the 2008–2009 Academic Year: Mechanism, Symptoms, and Management, William P. Meehan III, MD, Pierre d'Hemecourt, MD, and R. Dawn Comstock, PhD. The American Journal of Sports Medicine, August 17, 2010. 38: 2405–2409 (http://ajs.sagepub.com/content/early/2010/08/17/0363546510376737).

Impact of Playing Professional American Football on Long Term Brain Function. Amen DG, Newberg A, Thatcher R, Jin Y, Wu J, Keator D, Willeumier K. Journal of Neuropsychiatry and Clinical Neurosciences, J Neuropsychiatry Clin Neurosci 23:1, Winter 2011, 98–106. AB

Mechanisms of Head Injury, Alan R. Moritz. Boston, MA: Department of Legal Medicine, Harvard Medical School. *Annals of Surgery*, April 1943. 117(4):562–575 (http://www.ncbi.nlm.nih.gov/pmc/articles/PMC1617598/?page=1).

Mind and Brain: A Critical Appraisal of Cognitive Neuroscience, William R. Uttal. . Cambridge, MA: MIT Press, August 26, 2011.

Minimizing Concussion Isn't Cool Anymore, by E. Paul Zehr Ph.D. *Black Belt Brain*, May 12, 2014 (http://www.psychologytoday.com/blog/black-belt-brain/201405/minimizing-concussion-isn-t-cool-anymore).

NATA Issues New Position Statement on the Management of Sport Concussion, Steven P. Broglio, PhD, ATC*; Robert C. Cantu, MD†; Gerard A. Gioia, PhD‡; Kevin M. Guskiewicz, PhD, ATC, FNATA, FACSM§; Jeffrey Kutcher, MD*; Michael Palm, MBA, ATC‖; Tamara C. Valovich McLeod, PhD, ATC, FNATA. *Journal of Athletic Training*,

2014;49(2):245–265 doi: 10.4085/1062-6050-49.1.07 by the National Athletic Trainers' Association, Inc., (http://natajournals.org/doi/pdf/10.4085/1062-6050-49.1.07).

National Institute of Neurological Disorders and Stroke (NIH) http://science.education.nih.gov/supplements/nih4/self/guide/info-brain.htm

New Study Finds Concussion-Related Health Problems in Retired Football Players, Eurasia Review (http://www.eurasiareview.com/25022014-new-study-finds-concussion-related-health-problems-retired-football-players/).

Off-Season Doesn't Allow Brain to Recover from Football Hits, Study Says, *ScienceDaily*. University of Rochester Medical Center, 16 April 2014 (http://www.sciencedaily.com/releases/2014/04/140416172241.htm).

Pediatric Providers' Self-Reported Knowledge, Practices, and Attitudes About Concussion, Mark R. Zonfrillo, MD, MSCE; Christina L. Master, MD; Matthew F. Grady, MD; Flaura K. Winston, MD, PhD; James M. Callahan, MD; and Kristy B. Arbogast, PhD. Published online November 12, 2012, *Pediatrics*, Vol. 130 No. 6 December 1, 2012, pp. 1120–1125 (http://pediatrics.aappublications.org/content/130/6/1120.full).

Remarks by President Obama at the Safe Sports Concussion Summit, (http://www.whitehouse.gov/the-press-office/2014/05/29/remarks-president-healthy-kids-and-safe-sports-concussion-summit).

Reversing Brain Damage in Former NFL Players: Implications for TBI and Substance Abuse Rehabilitation, Amen DG, Wu JC, Taylor D, Willeumier K. Journal of Psychoactive Drugs, 43 (1), 2011 Online publication date: 08 April 2011 AB (http://www.amenclinics.com/dr-amen/latest-news/item/study-shows-reversing-brain-damage-among-nfl-players-is-possible-with-a-targeted-brain-healthy-protocol).

Sports concussion has long term impact on the brain, Deakin University, 16 December 2013 (http://www.deakin.edu.au/news/2013/161213sportsconcussion.php).

Sugar on the Brain, David DiSalvo. Forbes, 4/01/2012 (http://www.forbes.com/sites/daviddisalvo/2012/04/01/what-eating-too-much-sugar-does-to-your-brain/).

Sugar: A high-fat, refined sugar diet reduces hippocampal brain-derived neurotrophic factor, neuronal plasticity, and learning, Neuroscience. 2002;112(4):803–14. Molteni R1, Barnard RJ, Ying Z, Roberts CK, Gómez-Pinilla F.

Summary of evidence-based guideline update: Evaluation and management of concussion in sports, American Academy of Neurology (AAN), https://www.aan.com/uploadedFiles/Website Library Assets/Documents/3Practice Management/5Patient Resources/1For Your Patient/6 Sports Concussion Toolkit/guidelines.pdf

Teenagers Who Have Had a Concussion Also Have Higher Rates of Suicide Attempts, St. Michael's Hospital. ScienceDaily, April 15, 2014. http://www.sciencedaily.com/releases/2014/04/140415181325.htm

Teen Concussions Increase Risk of Depression, Health Behavior News Service, part of the Center for Advancing Health, Science Daily, January 9, 2014. http://www.sciencedaily.com/releases/2014/01/140109175502.htm

The Report to Congress on Mild Traumatic Brain Injury in the United States: Steps to Prevent a Serious Public Health Problem, Julie Louise Gerberding, M.D. M.P.H. September 2003, National Center for Injury Prevention and Control, part of the Centers for Disease Control and Prevention. http://www.cdc.gov/ncipc/pub-res/mtbi/mtbireport.pdf?utm source=Copy+of+Head+Injuries+Lead+To+This&utm campaign=BIA+2014&utm medium=email

Traumatic Brain Injury: Hope Through Research, prepared by Office of Communications and Public Liaison National Institute of Neurological Disorders and Stroke (NINDS). Bethesda, MD 20892, Accessed 4/30/2012, (http://www.ninds.nih.gov/disorders/tbi/tbi htr.pdf).

Traumatic Brain Injury Increases Risk of Parkinson's Disease, Mark Wheeler. UCLA News Room, August 19, 2011. http://newsroom.ucla.edu/releases/traumatic-brain-injury-a-threat-213647

Vascular Dementia, Lawrence Robison, Jocelyn Block, M.A., Melinda Smith, M.A., and Jeanne Segal, Ph.D. Helpguide.com, December 2014. http://www.helpguide.org/elder/vascular_dementia.htm

What is qEEG / Brain Mapping? (http://qeegsupport.com/what-is-qeeg-or-brain-mapping/?utm_source=Copy+of+Head+Injuries+Lead+To+This&utm_campaign=BIA+2014&utm_medium=email).

What We've Learned from Two Years of Tracking NFL Concussions, Jason M. Breslow, February 4, 2014. http://www.pbs.org/wgbh/pages/frontline/sports/concussion-watch/what-weve-learned-from-two-years-of-tracking-nfl-concussions/

APPENDICES

APPENDIX A

As Published in *Brain World Magazine*, Summer 2014

The Future of Sports Concussion Management

The prevalence of sports concussions, dangers associated with brain trauma, and related lawsuits escalating into multi-millions of dollars, are forcing athletes, parents, coaches and athletic trainers to reexamin4e their knowledge, protocols and culture protecting the players and games we love.

By Harry Kerasidis, M.D.

The brain is beautiful, the new frontier of science. But the brain is also vulnerable. It's buttery gel-like consistency floats unattached inside the skull. When force is applied, as it does many times in sports collisions, the brain sloshes from side to side, end to end, almost like scrambling an egg inside its shell.

The consequences can be seen immediately or take several minutes for symptoms to materialize. It's a mystery that science and the sports world are unraveling. They have to, because lives and futures are at stake, which until recently, have not been as important as wins and losses.

Athletes, young and old, are struggling with concussions and effects of mild traumatic brain injury. But the athletes aren't alone. Parents, coaches, athletic trainers, league officials, and virtually everybody else involved with supporting athletic development are grasping for answers to what can be done to assure athletes avoid the dangerous risk of short- and long-term cognitive and emotional impairment resulting from concussions.

Daily news report athletes suffering from concussions, the NFL and NHL are contending with multi-million dollar lawsuits because of related brain traumas, giving concussions an awareness level never seen before. While the Center for Disease Control (CDC) estimates more than 3 million concussions occur per year, most experts agree, the incidence rates are much higher than realized, since many athletes experience concussions more often than they actually report.

This has caused a rapid convergence of consensus statements and guidelines regarding the management of sport-related concussions to emerge, forcing the sports world to reexamine their knowledge about the brain and how to protect it, while allowing players to enjoy the benefits of the game, long after their playing days.

Unfortunately, parents and coaches aren't typically well versed in brain matters. And, the sports therapy and athletic trainer industries have been strapped with outdated learning, tools, and techniques. However, the time is now for technology and science to be combined, allowing integration of people and tools necessary for concussion clinical management at all levels and for all sports.

How Can Sports, at All Levels, Manage Concussions Moving Into the Future?

The phrase "concussion management" is still a relatively new concept leaving most sports teams with the task of piecing together various materials, tests, and tools to create protocols for managing concussions. These methods, which independently may be adequate to some degree, leave athletic trainers with a fragmented protocol that can delay, frustrate, and taint the objectivity needed to help prevent, detect, and protect athletes from significant brain damage. Therefore, a void has been created for a single, reliable, and practical protocol source of information that provides expert guidance.

I've been studying the brain for more than 25 years, treating thousands of concussions and specializing in the behavioral alterations associated with brain trauma. I found existing concussion management information lacks depth of understanding and realistic applications. So, I began creating my own protocols for education, baseline measurement, detection, and recovery guidance.

My conclusion is the sports world is starving to benefit from neurology and technology combining to create a seamless, thorough, and practical sports concussion management solution.

With the connectivity of the Internet, mobile applications, and advances with Information Technology, an end-to-end approach is now available to relieve the growing concern of athletes' brain health.

When referring to an "*hen referri solution*, I'm referring to a program that can be implemented for all sports and all levels from the beginning of the season to the end. This includes four key words in sport-related concussion management; recognize, report, recover, and responsibility.

Recognize

Provide proper awareness of the potential ravages of concussions, education that complies with state laws, and pre-season baseline testing that measures the full spectrum of cognitive and emotional performance tasks.

Report

Ability to immediately assess, document, and report results of post-concussion symptoms to necessary parties including the athlete, parents, coaching, and training staff, athletic trainers and athletic directors, medical professionals, and if necessary, league officials.

Recover

Guide the athlete and training staff through a progressive exertion protocol that helps determine when the athlete can be cleared for return to gameplay, as well as "return-to-learn" academic activities.

Responsibility

It takes a "team effort" to apply concussion management involving the athlete, parents, coach, training staff, medical professionals, referees, and league officials. The health of the athlete's short- and long-term future should weigh heavier than the desire to return to the field.

Internet-based computer technology offers a centralized method of accomplishing each of these steps in the process, and the ability to integrate everything into a single source, which has never been done before.

- Video training delivers online education on the proper concussion awareness for athletes, parents, coaches, and educators to optimize prevention, recognize the presence of concussion related symptoms, and encourage a cultural shift towards prioritizing brain health over gameplay.
- Smartphone technology is now at a level of sophistication to integrate assessment tools to assist responsible adults at the sidelines to document potential concussion incidents. This technology also allows injured players a convenient method of documenting concussion-related symptoms during the post-concussion recovery phase.
- The immediate connectivity of the Internet and email allows for instant alerts of potential concussion events to all key individuals involved in the athlete care. Athletic trainers and other healthcare providers can track injured athletes' recovery progress in real time, making post concussion management as efficient as possible. Reporting takes on other forms like a fully-integrated program. School administrators can instantly access data related to athletes and combined with parent-completed data, state-mandated preseason activities results, and school policies and procedures.
- A fully integrated computer-based system also allows for the objectivity and transparency needed to manage concussion properly under the watchful eyes of league officials and union administrators.

Research applications using a comprehensive, fully integrated computerized concussion-management system abound. For example, we could evaluate potential bio-markers to the vulnerability to concussion, identify the development of delayed effects of multiple brain trauma. Additionally, we could find clinical correlation of concussion incidence, and severity to bio-mechanical measures such as accelerometer technology, and the effects of therapeutic interventions on outcome measures such as recovery time and cognitive performance.

Retired athletes can also reap the benefits of a fully-integrated, computer-based system. Players who are cognitively asymptomatic can document their cognitive performance and experience of symptoms related to brain function online as part of a surveillance program meant for early detection and treatment of delayed effects of multiple brain trauma.

A complete concussion-management program as described gives the sports world a chance to have a "virtual neurologist" on its team, ultimately preserving the athletes health and optimizing their game performance.

# # #

Harry Kerasidis, M.D is the founder and medical director for XLNTbrain, LLC, based in Maryland, specializing in cognitive neurology. Through his practice treating hundreds of concussions, he created new baseline measures, assessments, reporting tools, and a 5-step recovery care plan.

APPENDIX B

As published on *PsychologyToday.com*:

Sports Concussion Psychology: Should We Take the Helmets OFF?

By Harry Kerasidis, M.D.

President Obama recently announced during a White House "Safe Sports Concussion Summit" that concussions are now a national priority. He said more research is needed, more awareness, better protocols, and better equipment. But what if safety equipment was contributing to the problem?

As absurd as this may sound, research suggests that this is a serious issue—the equipment designed to protect our athletes may, in fact, be weaponizing them and decreasing their sense of vulnerability.

It's a concept called "risk compensation" which suggests that people adjust their behavior in response to the perceived level of risk, becoming more careful when they sense greater risk and less careful if they feel more protected. Translation: If you wear safety equipment, you're inclined to take greater risk.

The theory emerged after several road safety interventions failed to meet expectations, and perhaps had the opposite effect. This "Peltzman Effect," named after Sam Peltzman, a professor of economics at the University of Chicago Booth School of Business, was reported in 1975 with controversy. Peltzman's study suggested increased highway safety regulation did not decrease highway deaths, saying "regulation was at best useless, at worst counterproductive."

More studies ensued in other applications, including:

- Cyclists wearing helmets rode faster, <u>Risk Analysis</u>,[13] 2011
- Drivers drive faster, less carefully wearing seat belts, <u>Accident Analysis and Prevention</u>,[14] 1994
- Condoms seem to foster disinhibition, <u>The Lancet</u>,[15] 2009

Football equipment has come a long way since it's rugby-like days in late 1860s, when some players strapped crude leather "head harnesses" around their head. Around 1905, mounting concerns about serious injuries occurring led many colleges to ban the game altogether. Then, President Theodore Roosevelt stepped in to help save the newly-loved game, forming what would become the National Collegiate Athletic Association (NCAA).

In the 1939, the NCAA required helmets, which the National Football League (NFL) followed suit in 1943, to reduce the risk of injury.

Today's American football players wear "Iron Man-like" armor, galvanized head to toe with thick synthetic materials. The shoulder pads stack 4 to 6 inches high, capable of absorbing—and delivering—enormous force. Helmets surround the skull snugly, protecting the skin and skull with virtually unbreakable polycarbonate alloy plastic, but surprisingly do little to protect the brain inside. Chest vests, appearing bullet-proof, cover the abdomen with extra protection.

Today's athletes are bigger, stronger, faster and have become finely-tuned collision machines capable of producing greater force than ever.

But would they hurl themselves with such abandon if they did not wear all the safety equipment, like rugby players?

While rugby and American football have evolved from a common past, the games have many differences including rules and equipment designed to protect the athletes.

---

[13] *Risk Compensation and Bicycle Helmets,* Ross Owen Phillips, Aslak Fyhri, and Fridulv Sagberg, (<u>http://www.cycle-helmets.com/P885.pdf</u>).

[14] *Seat-belt wearing and driving behavior: an instrumented-vehicle study,* W. Janssen. TNO Institute for Perception, DE Soesterberg, The Netherlands (<u>http://www.ncbi.nlm.nih.gov/pubmed/8198694?dopt=Abstract</u>).

[15] Ten myths and one truth about generalised HIV epidemics, James D Shelton, (http://www.thelancet.com/journals/lancet/article/PIIS0140-6736(07)61755-3/fulltext?_eventId=login).

According to Jim McKenna, a professor at Leeds Metropolitan University, (and a rugby coach) American football players often tackle head first, which is seldom seen in rugby. "Their head is the tip of the missile, with an enormous body of weight behind them," says McKenna. Meanwhile, the helmets and padding can actually make the situation worse, he thinks, encouraging them to use more force.

Maybe there's a safety lesson we can derive from rugby? Dr. Warren King, a team doctor for the Oakland Raiders and who has also worked with the U.S. National rugby team thinks so.

"I think the biggest thing football can learn from rugby is that, no, you can't use the head as a weapon," Dr. King said.

Rugby's contact rules are centered around the wrap tackle. A tackler can't slam into the ball carrier. He has to wrap his arms around and bring him to the ground. Tackling around the neck or head is illegal. Tackling low—around the ankles or knees—is fine, but because you have to wrap up, you're not barreling into a player, which leads to various injuries.

Without helmets (although some rugby players wear padded hats that are a little like football helmets from the 1920s), rugby players are taught from an early age to get their head to the side, and make contact with the shoulder.

Dr. King added that helmets are a double-edged sword as they can give an athlete a false sense of security (risk compensation) and risk of repetitive concussions remains despite the latest technology.

"We've learning more and more that these small concussions over time in a variety of sports can have a serious, lasting effect later in life," Dr. King said.

Safety gear may dull the impact to the body, but no equipment can dull the impact to the brain. No matter how much protection you add, there's no such thing as a "concussion-proof helmet." The brain was not meant to sustain the force caused by athletes crashing head-first into each other while wearing helmets and padding designed to absorb impact. Ironically, this equipment may put athletes' futures at greater risk.

It's a radical thought, but what if the game of football was to ban helmets altogether? John Tamny, reporting for *Forbes* agrees, writing in 2012 that, "if so, players will be far more careful about how they hit and tackle, and they'll do both with much less force."

Since the game itself has become more of a violent spectacle than athletic prowess, here are a few ideas to avoid risk compensation injury

Tips to Avoid Risk Compensation Injury

1. Educate parents, coaches and athletes about the risk compensation phenomena.
2. Safety gear is for protection, and does not make athletes invincible or allow them to take more risks or be more aggressive.
3. Teach proper, alternative tackling techniques, in football.
4. Increase enforcement of rules, or alter them, to reflect desire to protect athletes from brain injury.
5. Promote significant penalties for any "bounty" that encourages gladiator attitude to hurt an opponent.

#

Cognitive neurologist Harry Kerasidis, M.D. is the Founder of Chesapeake Neurology Associates in Maryland. He also serves as the Medical Director for the *Center for Neuroscience, Sleep Disorders Center* and *Stroke Center* at Calvert Memorial Hospital. For more than 25 years, Dr. Kerasidis has studied changes of the electrophysiology of the brain as it relates to behavior, cognitive function and emotional function resulting from various brain trauma, including concussions. His work led to the establishing the first complete concussion management program, xlntbrain.com.

APPENDIX C

An article as it appears on www.Naturallysavvy.com/[16]

Kids and Concussions What Every Mom, Coach and League Official Need To Know and Do

By Harry Kerasidis, M.D.

Sports provide an excellent platform to teach our youth about important, intangible life skills like teamwork, hard work, dedication, understanding roles, and overcoming adversity. All these life skills can be undone by injury to the brain due to concussion that is not managed properly.

Although concussions have caught the national media spotlight lately, most people—including parents, athletes, coaches, even medical personnel—have little respect for the consequences of concussion injury or know what to do when a hit to the head occurs. Whether it's during a contact sport or rough-housing around the home, concussions can have dire short- and long-term consequences if they are not treated carefully.

In my 25 years of studying the brain and behavior, treating hundreds of concussed patients, I've established a healthy respect for these traumatic events and hope to shed light on what every mom, dad, coach and league official need to know and do when they suspect a concussion has been suffered.

---

[16] Harry Kerasidis, M.D., *Kids Health and Concussions: What Every Mom, Coach and League Official Needs to Know and Do.* Naturally Savvy, March 13, 2014. http://naturallysavvy.com/care/kids-health-and-concussions-what-every-mom-coach-and-league-official-needs-to-know-and-do.

First, here's a little brain briefing:

1. **The brain is involved in everything.** Hand-eye coordination, memory, language processing, reasoning, decision-making, and emotional control are just the tip of the iceberg. The brain is critical to maintaining our health, behaviors and relationships.

2. **The brain is vulnerable.** The gelatin-like brain is highly sensitive, housed unattached inside a skull, floating in fluid. Helmets may protect the skull, but they cannot protect the brain from abrupt hits, whether they are head-to-head or hard falls. Even a whiplash event can cause physical and psychological brain trauma.

3. **The brain has many parts.** Each area or lobe, serves different functions. For example:

   - *Frontal lobes*: Executive processes, including control over emotional outflow, impulse control and focus, attention, planning, organizing, and decision-making.
   - *Temporal lobes*: Emotional and auditory processing, memory, and mood stability.
   - *Cerebellum*: Sensory interpretation involved with motor control, coordination, precision, and timing.
   - *Limbic System*: Emotional regulation, mood, motivation, and memory.

4. **A concussion is like a "brain sprain."** Like a muscle sprain, concussions vary in severity, from mild to moderate to severe with symptoms that are expected to recover in days, weeks, or sometimes months. A concussion is like a bruise to the brain, affecting the brain cells, or neurons, which result in obvious, and sometimes less obvious symptoms. Should symptoms continue beyond a few weeks, it is wise to see a neurologist for treatment of a possible traumatic brain injury. Concussion symptoms to look for include:

   - Dazed or vacant stare, confusion, loss of consciousness, amnesia, delayed verbal/motor response, headache, visual disturbances (light sensitivity, blurred or double vision), disorientation, inability to focus, nausea/vomiting, disequilibrium, mood swings, slurred/incoherent speech, excessive drowsiness or inability to sleep.

5. **Don't try to accelerate recovery from a brain sprain.** Don't let machismo toughness get in the way. If recovery from a concussion is not handled properly, it can cause permanent cognitive and psychological brain damage. Even worse, a concussion is most serious when a second concussion is sustained to an already injured brain, before the trauma has completely recovered. **This second-impact syndrome** may cause a sudden swelling of the brain, which can exacerbate the previous injury and even prove to be fatal.

Concussions don't have to kill contact sports, but moms, dads, and league coaches at all levels need to implement a "concussion management" protocol that guides them through the following:

Recognition

Every state in the U.S. requires high school and college sports teams to receive a certain amount of concussion education every year. The same should be mandated on the youth-league level. Additionally, every athlete should take a "baseline" test prior to the season, establishing normal cognitive and emotional measures for future comparison.

Reporting

Every sports team should enlist a "concussion coordinator" that has access to a sideline assessment tool, which guides them in the evaluation of the suspected concussed individual, recording symptoms, and reporting comparison scores to all involved parties. Athletes should be encouraged to report their own symptoms or signs of concussion in their teammates if present. Parents should be aware that often concussion symptoms appear hours or even days later.

Recovering

My biggest concern is an individual who returns to normal activity, even schoolwork or to game play too soon. Rest the brain and body, monitor symptoms daily, and use a progressive exertion recovery care plan to help establish when someone is ready to return.

Responsibility

Compliance and applying complete concussion management involves a community team effort. There needs to be a cultural shift towards prioritizing brain health over gameplay. Concussion knowledge contains the power to prevent, detect and protects our youth, giving them the opportunity to apply what they've learned on the field to real life.

Note to the reader: I created a concussion management system, called XLNTbrain Sport that provides each of the protocol elements mentioned in this article. Be a brain health advocate and share this article with your coach or league officials. It could the difference between a winning season and a winning life.

#

Harry Kerasidis, M.D., specializes in cognitive neurology. Through his practice treating hundreds of concussions, he created new baseline measures, assessments, reporting tools and a 5-step recovery care plan. Dr. Kerasidis also writes the "Brain Doctor Blog" to promote concussion awareness.

APPENDIX D

As published in Psychology Today:[17]

NFL Analyst, Players Point At Pride As Major Reason for Concussions

By Harry Kerasidis, M.D.

ESPN Football Analyst John Clayton recently said during Super Bowl week the biggest challenge with concussions is "players are always going to want to get back on the field as soon as possible." The toughness culture nurtures players' pride about their ability to sustain hard hits. It's this nature that is killing brain cells causing cognitive and emotional impairment and even lives.

But a "toughness" mindset is different than a tough brain. Clayton said even though scientists are studying concussions, and helmet manufacturers are advancing their protection, most people don't realize that all it takes is a hard fall to the ground.

"One dimension that rarely gets covered is the recoil effect on the brain," Clayton said. "It happens all the time, every game someone has one." However, not everyone reports concussion symptoms because of the toughness mindset.

---

[17] Harry Kerasidis, M.D., *NFL Analyst, Players Point At Pride As Major Reason for Concussions. Psychology Today,* March 31, 2014. https://www.psychologytoday.com/blog/brain-trauma/201403/nfl-players-say-pride-is-major-reason-concussions

"The NFL needs stronger protocols for how they handle it," Clayton said speaking of hard falls, hits, and the machismo preventing players from reporting concussions.

During Super Bowl week, many other former NFL players spoke about their experiences with concussions both on and off the field, including Percy Harvin, offensive standout for NFL Champions Seattle Seahawks.

After sustaining a hard hit in the NFC playoff game against the New Orleans Saints, Harvin walked off the field showing signs of concussion.

"I was dazed, but wanted to come back," Harvin said during the Super Bowl Media Day about that hit. "I was saying to myself 'how could this happen?'" Harvin had just returned after an 11-game recovery from a hip injury. But somehow, Harvin passed the sideline assessment and was allowed back into the game, and sustained another hit. This time, the concussion symptoms were more evident and he missed the rest of the game, and the following NFC Championship game against the 49ers.

Clinton Portis, former NFL running back said, during a C4CT Concussion Summit held at the United Nations in New York during Super Bowl week, that getting hit hard and getting back up is a matter of pride for players.

"The pride of being a running back was having pride in colliding with the other guy and hitting them as hard or harder than they hit you," Portis said. "But you don't realize how hard you were hit."

He is feeling the effects now. "I had a memory that was so crisp and now it's not as crisp as it was. My vision used to be one of my strengths, now it's not and I'm having migraines," said Portis, who played nine seasons in the NFL.

E. J. Henderson, a former NFL player, said he never had a medical diagnosis of a concussion, but during the game all players "remember those hits" that cause temporary concern. "Now I notice memory loss and a short-temper and I've only been out of the game for two years."

Robert Griffith, who played 13 seasons in the NFL, said his job playing strong safety was to be an "enforcer." In one game, Griffith said he told himself, "we are killing each other out here." Griffith said NFL players are often looked at as "heroes," but people need to realize concussions are making them "damaged goods."

"I think we all (former NFL players) have some short-term memory issues. I have to keep notes of everything and have my phone with me all the time," he said. "I now know the affects of the game because after four or five years, I began to see problems among players with sleep, depression, addiction, self-worth issues, and mood swings."

Lance Johnstone, played in the NFL for 11 seasons only missing nine games. He was also never medically diagnosed with a concussion. "But I can't tell you how many times I had to close one eye to see straight," Johnstone said. "As a player, you start to accept new norms of pain. Now I'm 40-years-old and I'm scared honestly. I have brain fogginess, a memory that things just slip my mind, and really have to concentrate in order to focus."

Isaiah Kacyvenski, who was a former seven-year linebacker in the NFL, said players become expert at playing with or hiding pain.

"The men who make it all the way to the NFL must become masters at masking pain," he said. "I never wanted to speak up about any issue I felt, particularly about concussions because they are known as 'unknown risk.'

After football, Kacyvenski earned an MBA from Harvard Business School, a seemingly impossible accomplishment after years of hard hits to the head.

"Losing focus is one of the most frustrating experiences," Kacyvenski said about his studying years. "I had to battle to get through school. Was I different after football? Unequivocally, YES."

It's time to re-define toughness in the game. While I believe mental and physical toughness to endure hardship are great assets, the brain physiology cannot cooperate. Perhaps we will see a new era in sports where toughness means having the humility to admit your brain is more important than the game.

# # #

Harry Kerasidis, M.D., is the founder and medical director for XLNTbrain, LLC, based in Maryland, specializing in cognitive neurology. Through his practice treating hundreds of concussions, he created new baseline measures, assessments, reporting tools and a 5-step recovery care plan, which he folded into XLNTbrain Sport™.

APPENDIX E

As published on PsychologyToday.com:[18]

Navigating the Most Serious Decision in Sports

By Harry Kerasidis, M.D.

The moment a jarring hit sloshes the brain against the inner table of the skull, the clock starts ticking. The next few minutes that follow lead to the most serious decision in sports. Because during this period, a number of neurological, physiological, financial, and perhaps philosophical, issues start bubbling to the surface, perhaps with life or death hanging in the balance.

Onlookers may be gasping or cheering with the sound of collision. Amidst opponent's trash-talking, teammates and coaches may be eagerly helping the player to his or her feet. The crowd roars with applause as the player walks off the field assisted by the athletic trainers. Is the cheering because the athlete is okay? Or is it because the player "took a hit for the team" and got back up? The athlete who sustained the hit immediately begins self-assessing their ability to return to play, tasking the potentially injured brain and body to cooperate almost instantly and signal a concussion pass or fail score.

---

[18] Harry Kerasidis, M.D., *Navigating The Most Serious Decision in Sports.* *Psychology Today*, May 2, 2014. https://www.psychologytoday.com/blog/brain-trauma/201405/navigating-the-most-serious-decision-in-sports

Unfortunately, the athlete is not the best judge in this decision. Nor are the coaches. Conflicts of interest abound. Hopefully, an athletic trainer or team doctor intervenes and carries out a series of tests to help identify the severity of a concussion risk.

Then, typically the decision is made—play or sit.

It's this period of time, from the hit to the return-to-play decision, where I fear sports may be risking too much. Too often, the post-hit evaluation process is rushed, with all eyes on the scoreboard, and not enough emphasis is on the future well being of the athlete.

Complicating matters further, signs of a concussion often take several minutes, hours, or even days, to materialize.

A concussion is considered to be a mild traumatic brain injury (mTBI). While science continues to discover ways of assessing concussions, numerous other studies show a connection between brain trauma and problematic futures. Consider these:

- Almost half of homeless men had traumatic brain injuries (http://www.sciencedaily.com/releases/2014/04/140425104714.htm).
- Teenagers who have had a concussion also have higher rates of suicide attempts (http://www.sciencedaily.com/releases/2014/04/140415181325.htm).
- Head injuries can make children loners (http://www.sciencedaily.com/releases/2014/04/140410083505.htm).
- Teen concussions increase risk of depression (http://www.sciencedaily.com/releases/2014/01/140109175502.htm).

Perhaps an even louder wake-up call is that most concussions are not reported, and overt concussions are not required to cause brain damage. A 2012 study by the *American Association of Neurological Surgeons*[19] looked at 45 high school varsity football players, none of whom experienced a clinical concussion during the season. The researchers concluded a single season of football play can produce measurable brain changes that have

---

[19] American Association of Neurological Surgeons (AANS). "Brain changes can result from participation in one year of contact sports, evidence shows." ScienceDaily. www.sciencedaily.com/releases/2014/04/140408154105.htm (accessed February 14, 2015).

been previously associated with mTBI—"adding to the increasing amounts of literature demonstrating that a season of participation in a contact sport can show changes in the brain in the absence of concussion or clinical findings."

Another grave concern is the condition known as Second Impact Syndrome, or sudden cerebral swelling that may occur when a second concussion occurs while the brain is recovering from injury. Most people don't realize the 50 percent fatality rate among individuals who suffer this fortunately rare event. Of the survivors, 100 percent will have permanent neurological impairments.

Then there is the more common Post-Concussion Syndrome (PCS). This constellation of symptoms, which includes migraine-like headaches, cognitive impairment, balance problems, sleep dysregulation and mood disorders can last days, weeks, months, or even years.

Is this brain damage avoidable? In theory, yes. Realistically, no. But risk can be mitigated. Some of us are trying to educate and implement interventions designed to make better post-hit decisions.

Here are a few pointers to help navigate the most serious decision in sports:

1. **Don't move the unconscious person**. In the event of loss of consciousness, don't attempt to move the unresponsive individual and risk exacerbating the problem of a neck and spinal cord injury. During a loss of consciousness, the brain and body are experiencing a forced re-boot, but the person's pulse and breathing should continue. Should the individual stay unconscious for longer than a minute, call for help.

2. **Better to wait, than be sorry.** A loss of consciousness may be the most obvious symptom, but also not likely to occur. Only one in 10 concussions result in a loss of consciousness. Therefore, onlookers have to be highly tuned into possible signs of a concussion. Symptoms can vary depending on the individual and where the brain suffers trauma. But generally, be aware of a glazed-over look in the eyes and perhaps signs of confusion within a few seconds.

   If there is any hint of this, I recommend asking the athlete if they can stand and walk or skate to the sideline unassisted.

Now, the waiting game begins. Give it at least two minutes before conducting any concussion assessments. Record and report the results and wait again. Don't let the athlete, or coach, try to talk themselves back into action.

I've created a protocol to help with the on-the-field concussion assessment. It involves cognitive, emotional, and balance measures using a mobile app, called the XLNTbrain Sideline Assessment Tool. This tool, a companion to the comprehensive XLNTbrain Sport™ concussion management program, guides the responsible person on the sideline through a step-by-step process of assessing memory, orientation, and balance for a potentially injured athlete and instantly documents and reports the results.

3. **Wait some more.** The least popular decision is to wait, perhaps another 30 minutes and conduct another concussion assessment. During this period of time, the brain is rapidly trying to heal itself, flooding blood and oxygen to the injury. Other functions may be compromised. Decision-making could be influenced. And further injury to the brain is the enemy, not the opponent on the field. Sometimes, concussion symptoms show up the next day. So, even if the athlete passes the sideline assessment, unless a trained medical professional has determined that there was no concussion, just the suspicion that a concussion may have occurred warrants that the player must sit out for the rest of the day.

4. **Allow for recovery** A recovery protocol needs to be set into motion. It begins with rest, minimizing mental, and physical stimulation until the athlete is symptom free. The concept is "relative rest," meaning the avoidance of any mental or physical activity that provokes the athlete's concussion-related symptoms. Once the injured player is free of symptoms at rest, I have included a 5-step progressive exertion recovery guide built into XLNTbrain Sport™ that monitors symptoms, and guides the timeline for a return to practice, or even classroom activities.

5. 5. **Decide**. Notice how careful I'm recommending a hard hit should be treated? A decision to allow a player to return to the game too soon, has too many risks. Give it time. Give it rest.

Follow a recovery protocol, monitor symptoms and then decide when to return.

The Public Broadcasting Service television program "Frontline" has been tracking concussions during the last two seasons of the National Football League (NFL). Among the alarming discoveries, 49.5 percent of players never missed a game after sustaining a concussion. Given that the average concussion injury taeks 10 to 14 days of recovery, I feel many of these players may be returning to the game too soon.

While there is no standard recovery time from a concussion, guidelines from the American Academy of Neurology and endorsed by the NFL Players Association, find that athletes are at greatest risk of repeat injury in the first 10 days post-concussion. And research suggests that the more head injuries a person suffers, the more likely they are to suffer from *chronic traumatic encephalopathy* (CTE) and face complications later in life.

The bottom line is that awareness and patience helps the athlete avoid becoming an unfortunate statistic.

# # #

Harry Kerasidis, M.D specializes in cognitive neurology. Through his practice treating hundreds of concussions, he created the, first and only, fully-integrated complete concussion management program that includes baseline measures, mobile assessments, reporting tools and a 5-step recovery care plan.

APPENDIX F

As published in *Athletic Business* Magazine

Taking Concussion Management to New Heights

By Harry Kerasidis, M.D.

Bravo, kudos, and applause are in order for the National Athletic Trainers' Association (NATA) for updating its "Position Statement: Management of Sports Concussion" from its original guidelines published in 2004. As sports programs across the country contend with the rapid convergence of concussion awareness, legal compliance, and risks associated with brain trauma, I applaud NATA for its intent to provide more comprehensive guidance.

I've personally suffered a sport-related concussion, and experienced the dizzying void of experienced guidance. The incident's after-affects of temporary memory loss and confusion, while otherwise fully-functional, compelled me to study the brain and become a neurologist. Since then, I've invested more than 25 years to understand the cognitive consequences from concussions, treating hundreds of concussed patients.

After reviewing NATA's new position, I'm glad they gave the topic its due attention. Based on my own experience and numerous cases I've personally attended to, along with the review of variety of opinions, and the science and understanding of concussions, I'm beginning to see areas in which concussion guidelines for any sports program can be enhanced. I'd like to share the following recommendations that complement the NATA guidelines both on and off the field.

1. Compliance Is the Key

It's one thing to establish a policy—or even a law, but it's another to follow it. Every state in the United States now has enacted student-athlete concussion-related laws. But who is monitoring? What are the repercussions for not following them?

Perhaps lives are at stake.

With so much on the line, the most important key to successfully protecting athletes from short- and possibly long-term brain damage is to establish and comply with a scientifically-based concussion management program.

Each organization needs to monitor its concussion management personnel like it monitors the bottom line. Typically, this would require having a single person responsible for the concussion protocols, providing some level of reporting for supervisory staff to review. Based on feedback, the protocols could be modified as needed. I recommend each sports program, even non-school sponsored programs, appoint a "Concussion Coordinator," who oversees the protocol the preseason process, ensuring proper equipment, education, and baseline testing. This individuals would also administer and report concussion-related activities. The Concussion Coordinator may be an athletic trainer or someone else affiliated with the program solely focused on the brain health of the athletes.

2. Establish Standards for *Methods*

Ask 10 doctors, get 10 answers. Unfortunately, concussions vary from person to person, and symptoms often materialize several hours or days afterwards. What is needed is a consistent application of methods for education, prevention, detection, and protection from concussions. The good news is that, through advances of medical science, there has been a convergence of guidelines for the management of sport concussion injury.

The lack of standardization of methods, however, has placed athletic trainers, or Concussion Coordinators, in difficult positions to decipher what should be implemented. And, I fear many athletic trainers still use outdated learning, tools, and techniques.

For example, in the area of education, almost every state requires parents and athletes to receive concussion awareness education. Often this is simply a printed sheet they have to sign before the athlete can play. In the end, how can we verify the parents and athletes *actually* read the forms they sign? How can we confirm the right people are receiving the right education and comprehending the material?

In the tool I helped create, an online educational activity covers the areas of concussion awareness that are necessary for adequate levels of education. Then, a quiz is required to be taken to demonstrate an acceptable level of understanding. The results are then available to be monitored.

The same goes with detection. There are a few telltale signs an athlete may be reeling from a concussion, like a dazed vacant stare or a wobbly walk. But after they've "shaken it off," what methods should be implemented to measure the severity of concussion, and help guide the decision about returning the athlete back to play?

Several tools, tests, and protocols are appearing on the market, leaving the Concussion Coordinator with the task of deciding what's best for their program. Therein lies the problem, because it's a monumental task of navigating the array of opinions and making quality informed decisions. "Best practices" for concussion management is still a moving target.

As a cognitive neurologist specializing in concussions, I assembled protocols and folded them into a fully integrated, comprehensive, clinical-caliber protocol for managing concussions. I've tapped technology to give athletic trainers and Concussion Coordinators a go-to, single resource that integrates recommendations from the best standards of care issued by the most respected organizations in the field: *NATA, the American Academy of Sports Medicine, American Academy of Neurology, American Academy of Pediatrics,* and the *International Conference on Concussion in Sport.*

My protocol covers the entire concussion management workflow from the beginning of the season to the end, including monitored educational activities, enhanced baseline testing, a sideline assessment mobile app that includes balance testing, post-injury symptom checking, and recovery guidance tracking balance, symptoms, and cognitive functions. This program integrates previously administered baseline test results with post-injury monitoring to establish the level of severity, risk and a recovery path and timeline.

3. "Return-to-Play" (RTP) Clearance Requires a Specialist

Concussion management is an emerging field. Many general practitioners and Emergency Room doctors are not fully aware of current concepts and guidelines to detect and manage concussions. But they can be.

A recent study measuring the "self-reported knowledge, practices, and attitudes about concussions," published in the *Pediatrics Journal* concluded the following:

> *Although pediatric primary care and emergency medicine providers regularly care for concussion patients, they may*
>
> *not have adequate training or infrastructure to systematically diagnose and manage these patients. Specific provider education, decision support tools, and patient information could help enhance and standardize concussion management.*[20]

Another study conducted by the University of Washington, highlighted the need for primary-care providers to seek concussion education and gain access to standardized guidelines to care for these athlete in the best possible way. Sara P. Chrisman, M.D., who led the study, concluded that laws requiring return-to-play decisions be made by medical personnel " . . . are not useful if clinicians do not recognize concussions or are

---

[20]   *Pediatric Providers' Self-Reported Knowledge, Practices, and Attitudes About Concussion,* Mark R. Zonfrillo, MD, MSCE; Christina L. Master, MD; Matthew F. Grady, MD; Flaura K. Winston, MD, PhD; James M. Callahan, MD; and Kristy B. Arbogast, PhD. American Academy of Pediatrics, July 11, 2012 (http://pediatrics.aappublications.org/content/130/6/1120.full.pdf).

unaware of RTP guidelines and allow athletes to return to play sooner than recommended."[21]

It's only logical that "Return-to-Play" decisions should be guided by medical personnel who are specially trained in concussion management. But I would add, clearance should be based on a multi-faceted evaluation of the concussed athlete, monitoring daily symptom checklists, balance, and neuro-cognitive testing. Although many primary-care physicians would not be considered "specialists," they can obtain this specialty training, which I've made available in my system to manage concussions properly.

Finally, I believe *every sports program*, and *every athlete*, should be required to receive concussion "baseline" assessments *every year*. I have many reasons for this, but the main thing to remember is that the brain changes over time, and events occur in the off-season that may affect an outdated baseline assessment.

While NATA has done an admirable job of updating its position on managing concussions, adding compliance monitoring, establishing standards for methodology and requiring enhanced education for those who provide RTP clearance, would take concussion management to the new heights.

# # #

Harry Kerasidis, M.D specializes in cognitive neurology. Through his practice treating hundreds of concussions, he created the, first and only, fully-integrated complete concussion management program that includes baseline measures, mobile assessments, reporting tools and a 5-step recovery care plan.

---

[21]   *Concussion Knowledge of Primary Care Doctors Falls Short, Study Says*, Lindsey Barton Straus. MomsTeam, 10/25/2011:17:45 (http://www. momsteam.com/health-safety/concussion-knowledge-primary-care-doctors-falls-short-study-says).

APPENDIX G

As published in *Athletic Business*:

Concussion Management Update:
3 Ways Contact Sports Should Embrace Head Hit Tracking

By Harry Kerasidis, MD

The Friday night-lights put the spotlight on the athletes on the gridiron. It's third and long, a passing down. The quarterback gets the ball off just in time. The receiver, the football, and the defensive back all converge at high speed. The sound of collision, helmet against helmet, can be heard from the top of the bleachers. The entire crowd— home and visitor— gasps. Then cheers come before anyone has ascertained that no injury has occurred. Fortunately, there is none . . . this time. Every hit counts. Every hit to the head can be one step closer to a breakdown in the brain. But for many in today's sports world, we wait until the damage is already done; intervening with a concussion protocol after the athlete shows obvious concussion symptoms.

Every team should have a concussion management protocol in place addressing compliant education, baseline testing, sideline assessment tools, symptom tracking, and return-to-play guidance. This should be a standard in sports. But, I believe an even higher standard is coming. Every contact sports team should embrace new technology that tracks the force and frequency of head hits using impact sensors.

Here are three areas where accelerometer technology can be used in conjunction with the concussion management protocol to protect athletes from brain damage:

1. Sideline monitoring of collision forces that may be sufficient to cause concussion.

Use of accelerometer technology from the sideline allows monitoring of collision forces that may be sufficient to cause concussion injury. Accelerometers can measure force of collision and rotational forces affecting the head, and so the brain. But there is a great deal of variability in vulnerability to concussion injury from one athlete to the next. Factors such as gender, size, history of migraines, and others may make one athlete exposed to a 90g force hit result in concussion while another receiving the same force remains standing, and ready for the next play.

While accelerometer technology will never replace human decision-making, the data can alert responsible sideline personnel when a player may have sustained a serious hit to the head, and may need attention.

Further research is necessary to identify the threshold level of force to be concerned about. Should we alert the sideline concussion coordinator when the force of the hit is 50G, 80G, 100G? Should thresholds be set lower for youth and secondary school athletes to more conservatively protect young developing brains? Should they be higher for professionals who are better able to consent to the risks of playing the sport?

Whatever the threshold, my protocol for integrating accelerometer technology into the my program is to pull any player who sustains a hit above threshold and assess them using the my Sideline Assessment Tool (SAT) which includes, coincidentally, accelerometer-based balance testing to look for signs of concussion. If the SAT is normal, the player may return to practice or gameplay under a watchful eye, since signs of concussion may be delayed. If signs of concussion are present, the player is removed and appropriate management protocol should be applied.

From a neurological perspective, it's the sub-concussive hits that scare me. We don't see them. Players don't know them. Coaches ignore them.

There is mounting evidence that sub-concussive hits may cumulatively contribute to brain injury and decreased performance on neuropsychological tests. Furthermore, increasing numbers of cases of Chronic Traumatic Encephalopathy (CTE) are being reported in athletes playing contact sports, who never had a "documented" concussion.

2. Hit Count monitoring for the cumulative effects of sub-concussive hits.

There is now a growing acceptance of the concept of the Hit Count, a term coined by Sports Legacy Institute (SLI). By counting and measuring the velocity of hits sustained to the head, we gain valuable data that can lead to preventing concussions and further brain damage.

Think of tracking hits and measuring impact velocity like baseball pitchers count their pitches. The more pitches, the greater risk of loss of control and potential injury. Likewise, the more head hits an athlete sustains, the greater the risk of short- and long-term consequences of repetitive brain trauma. Like the pitch count, impact sensors can identify how often athletes sustain possible sub-concussive hits.

At the summit conference hosted by SLI in 2013, a consensus was reached to set 20G force as the threshold for a sub-concussive hit. Here again, further research is required to determine how many and over what time period these hits can be tolerated. Until future research more accurately identifies these thresholds, I propose these thresholds be set to detect athletes that exceed the 99.9 percentile. This percentile would include the number of hits that athletes of comparable age, gender and level of play sustain over a week, a month, or a season of practice and gameplay. If any of these thresholds are exceeded, the athlete should repeat baseline testing to determine if these hits have cumulatively affected the player's brain function. If there is impairment over baseline, the athlete should go to relative rest until cognitive performance returns to baseline.

3. Monitoring to prevent re-injury during the recovery period after concussion.

Finally, accelerometer technology can be leveraged to protect our athletes' brains during the recovery phase after concussion injury. One of the key principles of concussion management is to protect the brain from further injury during recovery from concussion injury. At the same time, rehabilitation efforts call for increasing activity and progressive exertion as long as the symptoms of concussion are not provoked. Accelerometer technology can be applied, in this setting, by real-time monitoring of the recovering athlete during the progressive exertion phase of recovery to ensure that the level of exertion and contact during practice does not exceed normal expected forces.

One concern I have is the potential for an adverse response from young athletes. I can envision some players may adopt an attitude that they are going to "light up" their opponents helmet as a secondary goal to winning the game. Safe and effective implementation of accelerometer technology into a comprehensive sport concussion management program includes proper education, fostering a cultural shift to prioritize brain health, and safety over gameplay.

Merging hit count and collision force data improves athletic trainers and other "concussion coordinators" ability to detect concussion risk. It also presents an unprecedented opportunity to further research the correlations between traumatic forces to the head and clinical consequences, including duration and intensity of symptoms, impairment of cognitive performance and effects on balance.

In my own neurology practice, I've treated hundreds of concussed patients. Through my experience, I noticed a startling lack of clinical-caliber, yet easy to implement concussion protocols available on the market. So I developed XLNTbrain Sport™, an all-in-one concussion management protocol that includes the integration of impact sensors from GForceTracker, Inc. I would highly recommend investigating the merits of this system, as well as embrace the idea that every hit counts.

# # #

Cognitive neurologist and author Harry Kerasidis, M.D. owns Chesapeake Neurology Associates in Maryland and at Calvert Memorial Hospital, he serves as the Medical Director for the *Center for Neuroscience, Sleep Disorders Center* and *Stroke Center*. He writes for *Psychology Today* and his new book, "Concussionology: Redefining Sports Concussion Management" is due in 2015.

NOTE: Dr. Kerasidis sport concussion management system is a data collection tool and does not intend to diagnose, treat or otherwise suggest any other course of action that would substitute a certified medical professional. All participants should seek the advice of medical professionals for the diagnosis and treatment when necessary, including for final clearance or play.

APPENDIX H

Other news from <u>XLNTbrain.com</u>.[22]

XLNTbrain Dr. Harry Kerasidis Says Adding Marijuana Haze Doubtful to Help Concussion Daze

Concussion Expert Offers: 5 Best Practices to Recover from Concussions

NEW YORK, NY (January 30, 2014) — After reports that Commissioner Roger Goodell said the NFL would consider allowing athletes to use marijuana to treat concussions if medical experts deemed it a legitimate solution, Harry Kerasidis, M.D., medical director of <u>XLNTbrain, LLC</u> says there's not enough data showing a connection between using marijuana and aiding concussion recovery.

"When the brain is concussed, it's struggling to regain its chemistry and electrolyte balance, as well as repairing the cell membranes," said <u>Dr. Kerasidis</u>, who has treated hundreds of concussions over his 25 years studying the effects of concussions on cognitive behaviors. "Adding a substance that interferes with the repair and recovery process may have detrimental effects. Although the research suggests a neuro-protective effect of cannabinoid receptor activation in brain trauma induced inflammatory models, we are far from extrapolating that medical marijuana is a safe and effective method of treating humans with post-concussion syndrome."

Dr. Kerasidis is in New York this week introducing <u>XLNTbrain Sport</u>, the first complete concussion management program for all sports and levels

---

[22]   http://www.xlntbrain.com/press_releases/marijuana_haze

which includes a <u>5-Step Progressive Exertion</u> recovery plan to help guide athletic trainers and athletes back to normal activity and gameplay safely.

"Before prescribing medical marijuana for concussions, I'd need to see scientific double-blind, placebo-controlled studies measuring the short- and long-term recovery effects," said Kerasidis. "For concussion-related headaches, I suggest taking an anti-inflammatory agent, such as acetaminophen, until the athlete is symptom free. If the symptoms continue, then the athlete may have a mild traumatic brain injury requiring different treatment protocols that may include prescription drugs or nutraceuticals."

Top 5 Tips for Recovery from Concussion[23]

1. **Sleep** — Aim for 7 to 8 hours of sleep per night within the first week.

2. **Mental Rest** — Avoid strenuous mental activities to avoid provoking symptoms. Limit reading, writing, texting, using computer, and playing video games.

3. **Physical Rest** — Engage is no physical exercise until symptom free.

4. **Eat Healthy** — The brain needs a nutritional diet and perhaps some nutritional supplements, such as Omega 3 fatty acids, Vitamin B Complex, Vitamin E, and CoQ10 to enhance the healing process.

5. **Drink Water** — The brain needs water to facilitate returning to proper balance. Aim for 100 oz. per day.

Finally, Dr. Kerasidis says to avoid toxins, such as drinking alcohol, and smoking—"we are not yet sure where the marijuana comes in"—which can delay the healing process.

---

[23]   http://www.xlntbrain.com/press_releases/marijuana_haze

About XLNTbrain, LLC

XLNTbrain LLC provides the first complete sports concussion management program for all sports and levels. Based in National Harbor, Maryland, XLNTbrain assists health professionals with a fully-integrated concussion management program designed to help prevent, detect and protect concussions, guiding athletes safely back to normal activity and gameplay. More information is available at www.xlntbrain.com and by calling (855) 333-XLNT (9568). Media Contact: David Jahr, (949) 874-2667, david.jahr@xlntbrain.com.

# # #

APPENDIX I

Other News from <u>XLNTbrain.com</u>[24]

Cognitive neurologist Harry Kerasidis, MD debuts XLNTbrain™ at United Nations to distinguished audience, scientists

NATIONAL HARBOR, Maryland, (March 4, 2014) — As the sports world prepared for the Super Bowl, many of the greatest minds in sports concussions and brain trauma gathered to share the latest science, research and new products available to protect athletes from harm, during the #C4CT Concussion Summit. Among the expert panelists was cognitive neurologist Harry Kerasidis, M.D., who introduced XLNTbrain Sport™, the first complete concussion management program for all sports and levels, which was reported about on NFL.com that week.

Presenting at New York NFL.com that week, January 29, Dr. Kerasidis explained that technological advances, combined with his personal experience studying and treating hundreds of concussions, have formed a new clinical-caliber tool called XLNTbrain Sport™. Designed for athletic trainers, athletic directors, coaches, league official, and parents, XLNTbrain Sport™ delivers a comprehensive concussion management system. Comparative to the NFL's protocol, XLNTbrain is more suited for a wide range of sports leagues, schools and medical applications.

"It was an honor to be in such great company, all of whom are pioneering the new frontier of science -- understanding the brain, resulting impairment caused by concussions, and what is available to

---

[24]   http://www.xlntbrain.com/press_releases/cultural_shift

prevent brain-related traumas," said Dr. Kerasidis, a contributor to Dr. Oz's sharecare.com, is among an elite few neurologists in the world specializing in the impairment of cognitive and emotional performance resulting from concussions. "Perhaps more importantly, together we're fighting for a cultural shift in sports that puts the brain health and well-being of an athlete above wins and losses."

With Mississippi recently legislating concussion education, now all high schools and colleges in the US must face the cultural change that concussion awareness has brought.

"I think this is a huge step forward, however, the mandated legislation for concussion education could use a bit more accountability in most cases," said Dr. Kerasidis, referring to how the education is delivered and received. "Within XLNTbrain Sport™, we provide an online educational activity followed by a quiz, demonstrating the athlete, coach or athletic trainer has watched, listened and understands the material."

With more than 5,000 athletes currently using XLNTbrain Sport™, the cultural shift is beginning to become more evident both on the national awareness level and local practical level.

"We're seeing a gap between the need for education, and the need for concussion management application at all levels," he said. "Concussion management is not just baseline testing. It must include data management, reporting, and tracking of post concussion signs and symptoms. XLNTbrain™ fills that gap."

Among the subscription-based product highlights, XLNTbrain Sport™ provides online concussion education, baseline testing, assists with detecting concussions and guides athletes safely back to normal activity and gameplay.

More information is available at www.xlntbrain.com and by calling (855) 333-9568. Media Contact: David Jahr, (949) 874-2667, david.jahr@xlntbrain.com.

-end-

APPENDIX J

Other News from **XLNTbrain.com**[25]

New Xlntbrain™ Mobile App Demystifies Sports Concussion Detection with Sideline Assessment Tool, Total Program

XLNTbrain-Mobile Introduced As President Obama Hosts "White House Safe Sports Concussion Summit," May 29

NATIONAL HARBOR, Maryland (May 29, 2014) — The scary, mysterious moments after an athlete is knocked unconscious or stumbles to their feet after a hard hit to the head often leaves onlookers with many serious questions, and few answers. A new mobile application available today for free on Google Play, the XLNTbrain Sideline Assessment Tool™ helps demystify the concussion detection process with a simple, yet clinical-caliber ally.

The XLNTbrain-Mobile app introduction comes coincidentally with President Barack Obama's White House Safe Sports Concussion Summit, held on May 29.

In development for more than three years by cognitive neurologist Harry Kerasidis, M.D, the XLNTbrain-Mobile app guides athletic trainers, coaches, and team doctors through a series of cognitive and balance tests to help assess a potentially-injured athlete for concussion-related signs and symptoms.

---

[25]   http://blog.xlntbrain.com/new-mobile-app-simplifies-concussion-detection/

According to Kerasidis, XLNTbrain-Mobile is the first and only companion app on the market that seamlessly integrates with a comprehensive concussion management program. Called XLNTbrain Sport™, the program provides everything a sports organization needs to comply with statewide education requirements, conduct pre-season baseline testing, sideline assessments, recovery guidance, daily symptom tracking, and automated reporting available on a subscription basis.

"The app is used to provide a clinical-caliber concussion-risk assessment on the sideline or in the locker room, and includes a state-of-the-art balance test that utilizes the accelerometer technology built in to smartphones," said Dr. Kerasidis, a double board certified neurologist who has studied and treated hundreds of concussions in his 25-year practice. "But the real power comes when a sports team or organization taps into all the other modalities that I've incorporated into a single web-based resource."

XLNTbrain Sideline Assessment Tool™ features include (XLNTbrain-Mobile App):

- Documents time, date, sport, position, injury, observed, and reported symptoms
- Assesses word memory and orientation
- Delivers balance test using smartphone accelerometer technology
- Provides simple color code system (red, yellow, green) to assign possible level of risk
- Includes Glasgow Coma Scale and Cranial Nerve Assessment for medical personnel
- Sends email alerts to parents and designated healthcare professionals that a potential concussion has been recorded
- Results immediately available on the XLNTbrain.com dashboard
- Includes XLNTbrain Daily Symptom Checklist for injured athletes to track post-concussion progress

"Until now, coaches, athletic trainers, and other medical professionals have had to choose from a wide array of mobile apps and piece them together with various other protocols," said Dr. Kerasidis who is also the

Medical Director of the Center for Neuroscience at Calvert Memorial Hospital. "Now they have a single platform that meets and exceeds guidelines set by the National Athletic Trainers Association, the American Academy of Neurology, and other medical organizations and meets my clinical approval. It's like having a virtual neurologist on the sideline."

About XLNTbrain, LLC

XLNTbrain LLC provides the first complete concussion management program for all sports and levels. Based in National Harbor, Maryland, XLNTbrain assists parents, coaches, athletic trainers and health professionals with a fully-integrated platform designed to help recognize concussions, assist with detecting concussions and guide athletes safely back to normal activity and gameplay. More information about XLNTbrain Sport™ is available at xlntbrain.com, by calling (855) 333-9568 or emailing info@xlntbrain.com. Media Contact: David Jahr, (949) 874-2667, david.jahr@xlntbrain.com

# # #

NOTE: XLNTbrain LLC's sport concussion management system is a data collection tool and does not intend to diagnose, treat or otherwise suggest any other course of action that would substitute a certified medical professional. All participants should seek the advice of medical professionals for the diagnosis and treatment when necessary, including for final clearance or play.

APPENDIX K

Other News from <u>Xlntbrain.com</u>[26]

Gforcetracker™ Inc., Xlntbrain LLC Form Alliance to Introduce "Fully-Integrated" Sports Concussion Management System

New venture includes compliant education, baseline testing, impact sensors, sideline assessment, and post-concussion recovery guidance integrated into single platform

NATIONAL HARBOR, Maryland (June 24, 2014) — A new alliance formed between XLNTbrain LLC and GforceTracker™ Inc. (GFT) provides the first "fully-integrated" concussion management system to include Hit Count˚ Certified impact sensors with concussion management tools and software. Both companies will exhibit how the technologies have merged together for the first time at the National Athletic Trainers' Association (NATA) 65th Clinical Symposia & AT Expo at the Indiana Convention Center, June 25–28 (booth #206).

By integrating GFT's impact sensor technology into XLNTbrain's concussion management system, sports organizations can benefit from a single platform that meets or exceeds concussion protocols, guidelines and position statements established by NATA, National Football League, American Academy of Neurology and other medical organizations.

---

26   http://blog.xlntbrain.com/gforcetracker-inc-xlntbrain-llc-form-alliance-to-introduce-fully-integrated-sports-concussion-management-system/

The strategic alliance provides coaches, parents, athletic trainers and other medical professionals with a concussion management system that includes:

- Educational activity that complies with statewide sports concussion laws
- Comprehensive baseline testing
- Impact sensors tracking number and force of hits sustained by the head
- XLNTbrain-Mobile app that assesses and documents word memory, orientation and balance testing using smartphone accelerometer technology
- Email reporting to designated individuals
- XLNTbrain Daily Symptom Tracker tool
- 5-Step Progressive Exertion recovery care plan, guiding the return-to-play decision.
- A fully automated and customizable Return-to-Learn Academic Care Plan based on concussion symptoms to help injured athletes return to the school environment.
- XLNTbrain.com dashboard provides real-time monitoring of athletes in the system

"Merging hit count and collision force data through GFT impact sensors with XLNTbrain's technology improves athletic trainers and other 'concussion coordinators' ability of detecting concussion risk," said Harry Kerasidis, M.D., a double-board certified neurologist who has studied and treated hundreds of concussions in his 25 year practice. "While we await research and development announced recently through the White House, the most robust, clinical-caliber and fully-integrated concussion management system is available now. This alliance also presents an unprecedented opportunity to further research the correlations between traumatic forces to the head and clinical consequences, including duration and intensity of symptoms, impairment of cognitive performance and effects on balance."

Dr. Kerasidis explained a few ways GFT's impact sensors can assist athletic trainers with their concussion protocols both on and off the field because:

- GFT's accelerometers can detect force of impact, but athletes vulnerability to concussion injury vary given the same force.
- GFT's cloud-based software tracks sub-concussive hits which have cumulative toll on brain function.
- During post-concussion recovery, GFT's sensors assist with preventing re-injury to the brain.

Application Examples: GFT Integrated with XLNTbrain

1. GFT allows individual's to pre-set a maximum level of collision force. If an athlete sustains that force to the head during practice or gameplay, the player can be taken out for an evaluation using the XLNTbrain Sideline Assessment Tool. If there are no signs of concussion, the athlete can return to the game with close monitoring for the rest of the game and the days that follow.

2. If an athlete sustains a certain number of significant hits, the XLNTbrain Baseline Test can be repeated to make sure that these hits are not causing brain dysfunction.

3. While a recovering concussed athlete goes through XLNTbrain's 5-Step Progressive Exertion process, using the XLNTbrain Daily Symptom Checklist to monitor for recurrence of concussion related symptoms, GFT's real-time monitor ensures that the athlete's head does not experience collision force enough to delay recovery.

Paul Walker, GFT co-founder and President, said the alliance blends two technology systems into a single platform that delivers athletic trainers, athletes and sports organizations better data to make informed decisions.

"We are delivering the best in class, fully-integrated solution for sports concussion management,"eWalker added. "Combining the sophistication of our GFT hardware and cloud-based software solution, with the concussion management system of XLNTbrain we can now track impacts that accumulate over the course of a practice, game, season, year or lifetime and deliver evidence-based data that is highly relevant to to athletic trainers when conducting baseline testing and sideline assessments."

GForceTracker™ Inc. is the first sensor company to be Hit Count®nCertified for football, hockey and lacrosse by the Sports Legacy Institute (SLI). The SLI is a non-profit organization founded in 2007 by Dr. Robert Cantu and Christopher Nowinski to "solve the concussion crisis" by advancing the study, treatment, and prevention of the effects of brain trauma in athletes and other at-risk groups. Working with leading experts, SLI developed a lab-based test protocol that sensors must pass to be Hit Count®yCertified as well as a universal Hit Count® Threshold that all certified sensors use to begin counting hits.

About GForceTracker™ Inc.

GForceTracker™ Inc. is an advanced linear g-force and rotational impact sensor monitoring system that accumulates a lifetime of head impacts. The detection device monitors, measures and provides vital statistics such as number of impacts, severity of impacts, local alarming when the impact exceeds an acceptable threshold and accumulates this data to provide key metrics that determine whether its user has suffered a possible head injury. The GFT is currently the only Hit Count® Certified head impact sensor on the market and can be used by individual players or entire teams in both helmeted and non-helmeted sports. The GFT, which weighs less than an ounce, and is approximately the size of a domino can be attached to the outside or inside of the helmet, and can be purchased for individuals or team use. For more information please visit gforcetracker.com.

About XLNTbrain, LLC

XLNTbrain LLC provides the first complete concussion management program for all sports and levels. Based in National Harbor, Maryland, XLNTbrain assists parents, coaches, athletic trainers and health professionals with a fully-integrated platform designed to help recognize concussions, monitor hit count and severity, assist with detecting concussions and guide athletes safely back to normal activity and gameplay. More information about XLNTbrain Sport™ is available at xlntbrain.com, by calling (855) 333-9568 or emailing info@xlntbrain.com. Media Contact: David Jahr, (949) 874-2667, david.jahr@xlntbrain.com

# # #

NOTE: XLNTbrain LLC's sport concussion management system is a data collection tool and does not intend to diagnose, treat or otherwise suggest any other course of action that would substitute a certified medical professional. All participants should seek the advice of medical professionals for the diagnosis and treatment when necessary, including for final clearance or play.

APPENDIX L

About XLNTbrain, LLC

XLNTbrain LLC provides the first complete sports concussion management program for teams and individuals of all levels. Formed by investment partner Peak Neuro, Inc., XLNTbrain is based in Maryland where it has been beta-tested for more than three years with 5,000 athletes. The concussion protocol delivered is based on more than 25 years of studying the physiology of the brain and resulting behaviors caused from various stimuli and trauma. The brainchild of Harry Kerasidis, M.D., one of only few neurologists specializing in the impairment of cognitive and emotional performance related to concussions, XLNTbrain seeks to protect athletes from the dangerous consequences of undetected and untreated concussions.

Over his medical career, Dr. Kerasidis (aka: The Brain Doctor), has treated thousands of patients with concussions. Through his practice, he created new baseline measures, assessments, reporting tools, and a 5-step recovery care plan which provides the foundation of the XLNTbrain offerings now available anywhere, anytime through technological advances.

"In developing XLNTbrain, we took a step back and looked at concussion management from a clinical perspective and asked, 'What would be the best case scenario for sports teams,' said Dr. Kerasidis. We decided sports teams and athletes would benefit from having a virtual neurologist guiding them from end-to-end, so that's what we did with our online platform and mobile app. It's my 25-plus years of concussion experience packaged into one program that can be applied for an affordable annual subscription fee."

Recent NFL lawsuits and exploding consumer awareness of traumatic brain injury has motivated nearly all the states in the U.S. to establish concussion management law, mandating a certain amount of concussion management education. While these new laws have helped awareness, they have also revealed a gap in the sports teams' ability to adequately prevent, detect, and protect their athletes from concussions.

XLNTbrain fills that gap with the first complete concussion management program, assisting sports teams with a "clinical-caliber" program, that delivers everything the athletes and parents, team and league officials, as well as medical professionals need to comply with state laws, and provide the highest concussion care.

Delivered online and through a mobile app, subscribers to XLNTbrain receive access to a complete concussion management program designed to Recognize, Report, and Recover from concussions safely:

Recognize

Concussion Education: Online video training and completion quiz that complies with statewide regulations about causes, symptoms of concussion, and importance of correct concussion treatment.

Baseline Testing: A balance and web-based neuro-cognitive test developed by XLNTbrain LLC before the start of the season to create a baseline measurement of reaction time, attention, inhibition, impulsivity, memory, information processing efficiency, and executive function. The test also assesses mood, anxiety, stress and emotionality, a major distinguishing factor from all other sports concussion tools currently on the market. The results are then compared with the largest normative database of all these measures.

Report

Sideline Assessment Mobile App: Using a smartphone or tablet, concussion coordinators can now performs a series of sideline assessments, compare with baseline results, document the severity of concussion, guide on-the-field decision making regarding treatment and recovery time and report results via email to all-interested parties, including parents, coaches, training staff, and medical professional for further evaluation.

Recover

Recovery Care: XLNTbrain helps answer the most common question, "when can I play again?" Dr. Kerasidis created a tool that guides the decision-making process, giving all-involved individuals a recovery care plan that includes daily monitoring of symptoms, progressive physical, and cognitive exertion exercises and a timeline to safely return to gameplay.

ABOUT HARRY KERASIDIS, M.D.

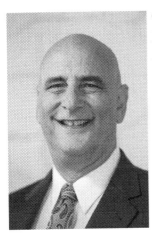

Cognitive neurologist Harry Kerasidis, M.D., has a distinguished career helping the public, scholars, and medical professionals understand the link between the physiology of the brain and behavior. He is the founder of **Chesapeake Neurology Associates** in Maryland and at **Calvert Memorial Hospital**, he serves as the medical director for the *Center for Neuroscience, Sleep Disorders Center* and *Stroke Center*. He is also a regular contributor to *Psychology Today* and *Athletic Business* magazines.

Known as the "Brain Doctor," Dr. Kerasidis is one of only a few elite neurologists in the world specializing in the impairment of cognitive and emotional performance resulting from concussions. He co-founded **XLNTbrain LLC** after 25 years studying the changes of the electrophysiology of the brain as it relates to behavior, cognitive function, and emotional function resulting from various brain trauma, including concussions.

Dr. Kerasidis has treated hundreds of concussion injuries in his practice as well as patients with a variety of cognitive and behavioral disorders including memory loss, sleep deprivation, ADD, dementia, Alzheimer's, and traumatic brain injury.

Through his experience, Dr. Kerasidis noticed existing concussion baseline testing lacked critical cognitive measures. So he created and began using his own baseline assessment, acute management, and recovery care plan, which has been incorporated into XLNTbrain Sport's complete concussion management program for all sports and levels.

- Chesapeake Neurology Associates—www.chesapeakeneurology.com
- Calvert Memorial Hospital — www.calverthospital.org
- XLNTbrain LLC — www.xlntbrain.com

Licensure

- Licensed to practice medicine in the States of Maryland, and Virginia.

Certifications

- American Board of Psychiatry and Neurology
- American Board of Sleep Medicine
- Diplomat, National Board of Medical Examiners
- Biofeedback International Certification Alliance

Professional Involvement

- American Academy of Neurology
- American Academy of Sleep Medicine
- International Society for Neuronal Regulation

Honors and Awards

- Hugh H. Hussey Award for excellence in teaching, 1990, as selected by the faculty of Georgetown University.

Education

A graduate of Georgetown University School of Medicine, Dr. Kerasidis completed his residency in Neurology and Fellowship in Clinical

Neurophysiology at the Georgetown University Hospital. Dr. Kerasidis' professional interests include cognitive neurology, sleep disorders, and behavioral correlations of EEG.

- **1992** Fellowship — *Clinical Neurophysiology, Georgetown University Department of Neurology*

    Training included clinical experience in epilepsy, including evaluation of medically refractory seizures for potential surgical intervention, intraoperative electrodiagnostic monitoring, evoked potentials, topographical mapping, electromyography, nerve conduction velocity studies, polysomnography and the diagnosis and treatment of sleep disorders.

- **1991** Residency — **Georgetown University Department of Neurology**

    Research: Four months research elective in basic neuroscience investigating the effects of levodopa on serotonin metabolism. Techniques acquired include stereotactic brain lesioning, high performance liquid chromatography, and data analysis. One year of research in cognitive evoked potentials in Temporal Lobe Epilepsy.

- **1988** Internship — *Georgetown University Transitional Internship*

    Curriculum: General Internal Medicine (four months), Pediatrics (four months), Emergency Medicine (two months), General Surgery (one month), Pediatric Neurology elective (one month).

- **1987 Doctor of Medicine**, Georgetown University School of Medicine

- **1982 Master of Science**, *Georgetown University Department of Physiology*, Research: Behavioral Assessment of Traumatic Spinal Cord Injury

- **1981 Bachelor of Science**, George Washington University

Teaching

- 1982–1983 Georgetown University School of Medicine — Teaching Assistant in Neurobiology.
- 1982 Georgetown School of Nursing — Teaching Fellowship, Human Biology, Anatomy, and Microbiology courses.
- 1979 George Washington University — Teaching Assistant in General Biology and comparative Anatomy.

Research and Published Studies

1. H. Kerasidis, K. Gale, J. R. Wrathall: **Spinal Cord Contusion in the Rat II: Behavioral Analysis of Functional Neurological Impairment.** Abstract presented at the annual meetings of the Society of Neuroscience, October 1994.
2. K. Gale, H. Kerasidis, J. R. Wrathall; Spinal Cord Contusion in the Rat: Behavioral Analysis of Functional Neurologic Impairment. Experimental Neurology, 88 (1985) 123–134.
3. H. Kerasidis, K. Gale, J. R. Wrathall; **Behavioral Assessment of Functional Deficit in Rats with Contusive Spinal Cord Injury.** Journal of Neuroscience Methods, 20 (1987) 167–189.
4. K. Kerasidis, P. Karstedt, R. Meloni, K. Gale, J. Pincus; **Effects of Levodopa of Regional Brain Metabolism in Rats with Unilateral Destruction of Dopamine Pathways.** Abstract presented at the annual meeting of the American Association of Neurologists, October 1990.
5. M. P. Kolsky, R. Packer, H. Kerasidis; **Miotic Pupils, Horizontal Gaze Palsy, Alternating Skew, Asymmetric Bobbing and Infiltrating Mononuclear Cells.** Abstract presented at the annual meeting of the Frank B. Walsh Society, February 1991.

INDEX

Printed in the United States
By Bookmasters